Gastric Band Hypnosis

Discover the Powerful Hypnotic Effect of Positive Affirmations

(Proven and Successful Meditation Techniques to Develop Healthy Eating Habits)

Edward McCane

I0136067

Published By **Darby Connor**

Edward McCane

Gastric Band Hypnosis: Discover the Powerful Hypnotic Effect of Positive Affirmations (Proven and Successful Meditation Techniques to Develop Healthy Eating Habits)

ISBN   978-1-7752672-3-2

No part of this guidebook shall be reproduced in any form without permission in writing from the publisher except in the case of brief quotations embodied in critical articles or reviews.

Legal & Disclaimer

The information contained in this ebook is not designed to replace or take the place of any form of medicine or professional medical advice. The information in this ebook has been provided for educational & entertainment purposes only.

The information contained in this book has been compiled from sources deemed reliable, and it is accurate to the best of the Author's knowledge; however, the Author cannot guarantee its accuracy and validity and cannot be held liable for any errors or omissions. Changes are periodically made to this book. You must consult your doctor or get professional medical advice before using any of the suggested remedies, techniques, or information in this book.

Upon using the information contained in this book, you agree to hold harmless the Author from and against any damages,

Table Of Contents

Chapter 1: Tough Loss

Why are you not able to lose weight

At a physical level, weight loss means eating less calories that you burn. However, the relationship between diet and weight maintenance is far more complicated than this. The cultural, psychological and medical factors that affect what you eat, how much, when and why, and how often, all play a major role in your diet. In this chapter we will review the main causes behind weight gain. We will address the key reasons behind weight gain, including:

* What: How does diet composition affect weight and health What foods are associated with weight gain?

* When: What does eating when affect your weight? How do habits and routines in eating lead to unhealthy eating habits?

* Why: How do cultural and psychological motivations and associations to food and the act eating influence your weight? We'll examine the reasons that you might be inclined to eat more calories than you need.

* How: How do you eat and choose to eat, and how does this interact with your emotions so that binging can be induced? How can sugar addiction result from sugary food and emotional factors?

Furthermore, we will present a clear, concise description of how a healthy and satisfying relationship with food is. This information will allow you to be more confident in your ability to apply it and identify the causes of weight loss.

Beware of the Misconceptions Around Weight Loss

There are two common misconceptions about weight loss. In this chapter, you will have to identify which misconceptions are affecting you and in what ways. These misconceptions stem from misunderstanding the concepts of healthy food, losing weight, and eating well. They may include beliefs or assumptions like:

Losing weight should not be difficult. People will give up on exercising and dieting if the process becomes too difficult. Weight loss can be achieved through regaining nutrient and fat-burning balance, hormonal balance, recovery, and the development of a realistic and sustainable exercise schedule. It is a process of changing your lifestyle. It isn't easy nor quick. For weight loss to occur, it takes patience, self assessment, tracking, trial and error, and persistence.

There is not one right diet. People try to lose weight by looking for diets that work. They don't realize that everyone is different. Each person's body type, weight, metabolism, hormonal state, lifestyle, etc. all have an impact on their nutritional needs. Without a proper understanding of your nutritional needs, even the best and most satisfying diets will not help you lose weight.

5 Main Reasons That You Aren't Losing Weight

Other than food itself, many factors affect your relationship with food. Your environment's food culture and your beliefs about food and food are key factors in determining what and how much you eat. Eating is not just about keeping your body functioning. Food is an integral part of our psychological, emotional and spiritual lives. We associate eating with pleasure and ease, reward, or celebration. But we also associate it as guilt and shame. The following are the biggest influences on your relationship to food:

Food and culture

Culturally positive associations with food can be made because it is used as an incentive for good behavior or achievement. This is fine as long the food does not become the main or only means of rewarding yourself, celebrating, or providing comfort and ease.

But many childhood associations with food can lead to negative feelings that can be hard to shake. For a parent, emptying the plates is the greatest daily achievement. It ensures that a child has enough food and is comfortable. The parent also feels fulfilled knowing that they did their job properly. It is important that their children enjoy the cooking they make. Ideal relationships with food are formed through playfulness and mindfulness, creativity, imagination, and explorations of different tastes, textures, flavors, and colors. This helps the child to develop neurophysiological skills and become more comfortable with the act of tasting and eating new foods.

Parents are often alarmed when their child won't eat due to unfamiliar flavors or overwhelming tastes, or because they don't want to eat. They fear that their child won't get enough nutrition, and they may end up getting sick. In these cases, parents may resort to:

* Guilt ("You're eating food that isn't needed when there are so many hungry kids out there!"

* Shame

* Threats

* Emotional bribery ("Eat up! Show me how much your love!"/"I love you more when it's you that eats than when you don't."

A child may not feel hungry. Children may have a lower need for food than many adults assume. But they often eat because they feel inadequate if it isn't.

This feeling follows them through adulthood. Gradually, they start to eat to either reward themselves for hard work or find consolation in bad moods, entertain themselves when bored, or just to acknowledge the fact that there is food in a world with many hungry people. These motivations make it harder to see the difference between what you think you should have and your true hunger. It is up to you, as a person, to determine how much, when and what. Gradually, this can lead to weight gain. You eat what you think you should versus what you actually need.

It only takes 100 calories more each day, which is just enough for a snack, to gain over 20lbs in a span of 10 years (Kaye und al., 1988).

If you have trouble losing weight, it is likely that you are eating a lot and not enough. It could be cultural or family-based eating habits. In this way, weight loss involves changing the way you think about food and how you eat it. To begin uncovering these influences, ask yourself the following questions.

* What lessons were your parents/caregivers teaching you about food. Did you feel guilty or ashamed about eating the food your parents prepared? Did you fear that you might get sick if there was not enough food on your plate?

* What's the food culture in your environment? Is there a requirement to eat even if you don't feel hungry, in order to honor the host and the occasion? If you're expected to eat together with your friends, then saying "no" would be considered offensive. The cultural influences on eating will influence your social relationships. This will help to avoid eating out for social reasons and allow you to have more meaningful conversations.

* How does food affect your life? Consider how much food you eat for hunger, and how much you eat habitually or out of love with food. Do you have a routine of making breakfast every morning? Do you indulge in eating every night while watching TV or movies to unwind after a hard week?

* What should your diet include? Is unhealthy food a common problem? Is it the inability to shop for healthy foods? Or do you cook with extra oil or fat to speed the process up? Do you eat to soothe your emotions? Do you feel hungry if you're upset and angry? Do you feel hungry when you're angry and upset?

These questions will help answer your family's, cultural, or personal questions about how they affect your weight and diet. You will be able to recognize when it is okay to eat. This is the first stage of changing your relationship and perception of food.

Food and Emotions

The next step in changing how you relate to food is to investigate emotional components (Geliebter, Aversa and 2003). Anxiety can be severely affected by stress, frustrations, sadness, and depression. Stress, anxiety, panicking and other stressful situations can cause your body to release sugar from the blood. This causes you to crave more sugary food in order compensate. Hormonal balance or, to be more precise, imbalance is another way your moods impact your appetite.

When you're feeling anxious, sad, or stressed, your blood levels increase (Francois and al., 2015.).

These hormones activate instinctive reactions when there is danger or threat. Your metabolism slows down when these hormones are present. You see, all of our primitive neurophysiological functions are designed to allow us to survive in hostile conditions. Your body will react to stress from work problems and relationship issues as if there is imminent starvation. Remember that the human race was born in an environment of food shortages. Any kind of threat, such as a fire or being chased down by a wild animal meant that you had to exhaust precious energy sources. A primal human would need to be nourished if this threat continued.

Our "defense systems" then slow down the metabolism to ensure survival. Although primal humans were far more active than today's, they used a lot of calories and burned a lot more calories than modern humans, who move a lot less. In such situations, where there's a lot to eat, as well as a lot more stress and less physical activity, our natural mechanisms can be prone for fat storage. They perceive constant danger (hypothetical threats can be detected as real) as well as an increase in appetite just by being around food. The relationship we have with food becomes more habitual and unconscious due to cultural and emotional factors. In reality, we actually need much less food than what we think, especially for those who have a nine-to-5 job.

The mental shift required to reframe how you relate to food involves redefining your perspectives on life. To do this, you can re-examine your stress triggers. Ask the following questions.

* What did I feel before becoming suddenly hungry?

* What was my pre-eating thought?

* What about the situation that triggered my craving for food?

These questions will help you identify the thoughts and emotions that drove your sudden craving for food. These insights can help you question your next cravings before you decide whether or no to eat.

The act of suppressing your feelings can result in emotional and unconscious eating. Because we are afraid of causing more pain than our bodies can handle, many people don't think about the things that really concern them. This isn't true.

Let's pretend you were asked to identify all situations which caused stress and subsequently the urge to overeat. What were these situations? What feelings did they trigger? Is it possible that you felt shameful or inadequate at work because of a coworker's comment about how late your report was? Or you were told that a coworker had gotten engaged. Which could have added to your feeling of loneliness, mistrust, and inability to find love after a hard breakup.

The best way to reduce stress is to break down these situations and change the way that you think about them. One example is if you tend to make assumptions about why people behave a certain way. It can lead you to believe that people see you negatively, or that they are malicious. But their reactions could simply be because of their own frustrations and insecurity. The best way to relieve stress is to not think that someone dislikes or treats you poorly because they act rudely.

Sadness can be difficult to cope with. A feeling of sadness caused by loss can lead to an illusion that allowing difficult emotions to surface will cause overwhelming grief. It won't. It is quite common for people not to feel contented by the pleasure of eating sugary sweets or other sweets. (Spence 2017. These foods are good for your serotonin levels. This hormone is responsible to bringing you happiness. You can stimulate serotonin via healthier activities, such as walking in nature and a conversion with an open-minded friend. Art, reading, self care, and self nurturing can all help boost serotonin levels. Re-shaping your response to sadness can be done by looking into the emotions caused by loss and then reviving moments when you were happy and fulfilled.

Exercising and watching movies can help you temporarily get over sadness, such as if your ex-partner is missing you or the loss you suffered. The sadness will return, so it's important to practice a better response.

You may experience emotional cravings and binging when you are dealing with grief, failures at the workplace, or temporary losses in a loved one.

Let's say that you have made an error at your job and your superior brought this to your attention. Perhaps you feel like a failure and are sad that your hard efforts aren't paying off. You might be tempted to order take-out, binge-watch your favourite TV show, or simply to eat junk food. Let's explore other ways of dealing with this. Instead of eating, think about how the events at work have made you feel.

* Did someone say something that made you feel unworthy or like a failure.

* Is this a negative event that has any consequences for your career?

* Is the situation really as bad and dire as it appears?

This analysis may lead you to the conclusion that you might have exaggerated your chances of a negative outcome. If you didn't find your work useful or needed within the company, why would they continue to employ you? Now it is time to recall some of the positive memories you have that may help you feel better, and resist the urge to eat.

* You can probably remember doing a great job, feeling validated and appreciated, and feeling empowered.

* Take note of at most three instances where your talents, engagement and contributions have been helpful to the organization. Particularly, remember all the times you helped your coworkers even though it wasn't required or asked for. It's not uncommon for employees to do these things at work. Even if you don't notice it, you are the one who should.

* Keep in mind your successes, charity work, and small acts for kindness that you did for others around you, such as family members, friends, and

colleagues. You will be a happier person because of these positive experiences.

* As you reflect on the pleasant memories, you should ask yourself what actions and events reveal something about you. What do you think that if you gave your all, worked honestly and with integrity for the organization, does that tell you about you? I believe that you are a caring, talented, creative, hardworking and caring person.

* Take the time to write down the useful labels, and then take as much time as needed to notice the positives.

If you want to take this happy experience and turn it into positive experiences, you can write down how the person you describe would respond in stressful situations. You may be able to show more patience and calm down before reacting with anger. Or you might want to slow down and consider how much of the frustration experienced by another person was caused or contributed to their stress, tiredness, overwhelm, and other factors.

It is hard to handle anger and hostility. So people choose to either lash out or suppress their feelings. Both are not helpful and often cause overeating. If you engage in an argument, you'll feel down and want sugar to lift you spirits. You can keep your anger at bay to avoid confrontation.

Instead, learn to react in a more assertive and fact-focused fashion. Finally, remember how you are a compassionate, caring, creative, and compassionate person. If you are confronted with difficult people, assertiveness means responding to the facts rather than their tone and bodylanguage.

Example

Your boss might be screaming at you, abusing authority, or criticizing an error you may have made. You can't respond to your boss's anger by suppressing your anger. Instead, acknowledge that you are angry and release it by deep, even breathing. Your boss may ask you what you should do to fix the problem or repair it. Your goal is to get to the bottom of the matter.

It is possible to make a mistake at work and fix it. Your anger will diminish as the conversation shifts to a more measured tone. Now, instead of dwelling on how hostile or dislikeable your boss might be, think about the actions you'll take to improve and correct your work.

Once the event is over, think back to the lessons it taught. How can you make the most of the experience to improve your work habits, communication, and behavior? Take a few minutes to write down your ideas and you will be calmer. Regular practice will reduce stress's power and help you develop a routine of healthy emotional processing.

Self-Image

Self-image can be defined as a set of beliefs about self worth, beauty, competence, value, and worthiness. Obesity can also be associated with negative thoughts about yourself such as believing you are unattractive or unworthy of love. Body image is directly related to self-image and what you believe about yourself (Hilbert-Caffier and Tuschen–Caffier, 2004). This can cause you to gain weight or maintain excess weight by not loving and respecting your body in its entirety.

If you don't believe that you can lose weight and think you're unattractive or lazy, you will unconsciously choose unhealthy foods. It can also hinder your ability and motivation to get healthy. It can create feelings of shame, awkwardness and guilt towards your body. This can lead you to avoid exercising or feel sluggish and tired right before the exercise. If you have a negative self image, your mind will try to protect itself from the judgement and scrutiny of others. This can result in unhealthy behaviors like binging and sleeping late, not exercising enough, and making it hard to try healthier foods.

Relationship with Physical Movement

You self-image and your relationship with movement are directly affected by the things you learned about yourself as a kid. Children who are encouraged and motivated to attempt and fail in sports rather than being criticized and scrutinized for them succeed more often and become healthier, more fit and more sport-oriented adults.

People who are teased for their inability to do sports or fall or for being tripped up or fallen often feel ashamed of their bodies. "Movement blockages" occur when people are unable to move, train, dance or dance. These blocks are designed to stop difficult memories from developing that can be associated with movement. They cause stiffness, unbalanced, and disorientation when working out. Movement blockages can be overcome using a gentle approach. Choose activities that bring you joy, like dancing, Qi Gongs, hiking, swimming, and yoga. You should also question your beliefs about your physical ability and examine them.

Understanding of Nutrition

In order to provide adequate nutrition, the body must have a good balance of macronutrients and micronutrients. This will allow it to burn fat and fuel its functions effectively. This balance is not universal.

The recommended macronutrients ratio amounts to around 40% carbohydrates and 25% fiber and protein (Simpson 2015).

The amount of food you eat will be determined by your health, movements, and current calorie intake. How to choose the right diet for your nutritional needs

* How many calories do you burn each day?

* Calculate your recommended food size.

* Understanding the macronutrient ratios of different foods.

Chapter 2: How Do I Feel Hungry

This chapter will provide information about your digestive system. You will learn the reasons you feel hungry, as well as the biological mechanisms. Also, you'll learn more about the biology behind weight gain, why it is so hard to lose weight, and what you could do to combat these problems.

How Your Digestive System Works

Your digestive process processes food so that valuable nutrients travel from your mouth and into your bloodstream. By doing this, your body gets the nutrients it needs to convert them into energy. Your digestive system is comprised of:

* The gastrointestinal track. Your gastrointestinal tract comprises multiple organs. They run from your mouth up to your anus. It contains your

mouth, stomach and large and small intestines, along with your anus. These organs can be hollow or joined together. The small intestine includes the appendix (cecum), colon, and rectum. Your appendix is an organ in the pouch that attaches to your cecum. Your colon connects to the large intestinale.

* Liver

* Pancreas

* Gallbladder

* Gut bacteria is an ecosystem made up of bacteria living in the gastrointestinal track. It breaks down nutrients and passes them into the bloodstream. Additionally, it synthesizes important nutrients like iron and vitamin k. Your digestive system and your blood, circulation, hormones and nervous system work together to process the foods you ingest.

Digestion is an important biological function because it allows food nutrients to be absorbed. These foods serve as energy for the body's function and regeneration of cells and tissues. You eat proteins as amino acids and fats as glycerol/fatty acids. Carbohydrates then become sugars. Ingestion of food will cause it to be broken down into smaller pieces, which are easier for the cells and tissues to absorb. The large intestine absorbs water from the foods you consume. Undigested parts of food are ejected.

Both hormones, nerves, and other chemicals are involved in the functioning of your digestive system. Peristalsis happens when you ingest foods. This is where the hollow organs of your gastrointestinal tract contract and relax to allow the contents to flow through the entire system. First, chew food with your tongue. This softens the foods and allows digestive juices, such as stomach acids and enzymes to break them down to form molecules that can then be processed.

Your pancreas creates the enzymes that breakdown macronutrients. This enzyme is then transported into the small digestive tract via small tubes, which connect the gland with the small intestine. Your liver is responsible to digest vitamins and other fats. It produces bile. This travels through ducts and from the liver into the gallbladder to the small intestine.

The Hunger Biology - Ghrelin and Leptin Hormones

It could be that even though you ate less than an hour ago, you still feel hungry. Why is this so? Hunger is a biological, psychological, and psychological sensation. It serves one purpose. It tells you to eat to fuel your body and make it function. But is this biological hunger, or psychological hunger?

In a world of constant food, it is difficult to differentiate between true and emotional hunger. Hunger is an evolutionary concept that reminds us when it's time for us to eat. Sometimes hunger can manifest even when there is no need to eat. This is due to the way our brains wired to seek out food. Nowadays food is easily found all around us and we don't have to search far to find it. However, this wasn't always the case. Primal humans had the need to work extremely hard to get food. They had to climb trees to collect food and hunt for nutrients. From the dawn of humanity, we were an Omnivorous species. That means that our ancestors consumed a wide variety of food.

The fear of running out was what caused early humans to eat. While our brains may have developed and evolved into more complex functions over time, some primal instincts still remain. Because modern life can consume one's attention to the point that they don't feel hungry, it is understandable. Our brains will often be drawn to foods rich in protein and fat. These are the essential nutrients that keep cells and tissue alive.

After finishing a meal, your stomach slowly empties itself by pushing the food through the system. Once this is complete, the so called migrating motor compound picks up any food that hasn't been fully digested. This takes about an half hour. After this, the hormone Motilin induces a growing sensation in the stomach.

Ghrelin, on other hand, is another hormone involved in hunger. It activates the hypothalamus neuronal network, which sends hunger signals. The hypothalamus' neurons control hunger. If the neurons in your hypothalamus are stimulated, then you will feel hungry. You can still feel hungry after meals.

Hunger can be either hedonic, or homeostatic. The first is biological and is connected to a biological need. The second type can strike when we are sad, bored, nervous or overstimulated. Hedonic hunger is better understood than biological hunger. Some of it has to do with the possibility to feed ourselves additional foods even when our stomachs feel full.

It also depends on how satisfied you are with your previous meal. If you feel hungry or don't like what you ate, you may look into additional foods.

What Happens If You Are Overeating?

Your brain monitors your hunger levels based on signals that indicate whether you are satisfied. There are many levels of feeling satisfied or full, and these feelings don't always correlate with biological grounds. Hunger can be profoundly emotional. You may eat large quantities of food and not feel full. Instinctively, we will strive to supply more calories when possible. While this strategy was effective in food shortages, it can lead to obesity and overeating. As you know, we live in an environment that offers a wide variety of foods. This makes us less active and more like our ancestors.

Furthermore, our foods are chemically more diverse than organic and natural. The majority of foods we eat today contain at least some chemicals. Overeating can also be affected by these chemicals as they alter the hormonal balance of the human body.

You can see that hunger doesn't always relate to physical hunger. It may also be related to cultural, psychological, as well as chemical influences that influence your gastrointestinal system. An inability to eat or see food can lead to a feeling of hunger. Even just thinking about food can cause hunger. Your body has its biological rhythm. This inner rhythm is related to your body's biological functions and hormones. It can lead to feeling hungry when you don't really need it.

Your body signals your brain to tell you when you feel hungry. Your brain signals this to your body so that you can replenish your food supply. When your stomach is empty, for longer than 2 hours, it contracts to allow the stomach to take in food and get into your intestines. This process is called "borborygmus" and can also be known as "stomach noise". Ghrelin levels in obese individuals are typically higher.

Yet, the levels of nutrients in your body, including fatty acids as well as amino acids and glucose, are very low. This signal tells us to eat. Hunger isn't just biological. It can also cause psychological problems. It will make it harder for you to concentrate and make decision. Feeling too hungry can make you feel physically sick.

Ghrelin does not just relate to homeostatic food. Ghrelin has a lot of things to do with hedonic or hedonistic eating, particularly as it mediates some stress responses. Ghrelin, in addition to controlling hunger, also has numerous anti-aging effects, such as cardiovascular and metabolic ones. Ghrelin levels will vary depending on how you eat. Ghrelin is also linked to eating habits. However, it was found ghrelin levels were lower in obese than overweight women.

Ghrelin levels are affected by total calories consumed. Higher calorie intake is associated with higher levels of ghrelin, although this does not apply to the obese. Ghrelin is not linked to heart rate, bloodpressure, or insulin resistance in obese individuals. The measure that correlates hedonic or stress eating is called the "total plasma Ghrelin" and it decreases with obesity. Ghrelin may have contributed in some cases to obesity, even though its primary function was to prevent hunger.

Ghrelin, which is a 28-amino-acid protein, is produced in the stomach. GHSR, or growth hormone secretagogue receptor, is one receptor that this hormone interacts with. GHSR and the hormone can be found in various parts of the body. This hormone is secreted into the stomach mucosa whenever energy supplies run low. It signals the hypothalamus by stimulating the vagal nervous system. This increases appetite and therefore, food intake. After eating, plasma levels are reduced.

Ghrelin and hedonic binging can be explained by the system of food induced reward. One will be more inclined to eat after eating and have a greater preference for sweets if they have high levels of Ghrelin. This is a clear indication that ghrelin could cause hedonic or compulsion eating, even though it's not necessary.

The stress response is also linked to ghrelin, according to scientific evidence. It was well-known that chronic stress sufferers are more likely than others to overeat or resort to comfort food. We now know that the hormone "ghrelin" mediates this phenomenon. Like the examples above, it has been shown that obesity increases the response. People who are lean have the highest levels ghrelin. Ghrelin is associated with increased blood glucose, insulin resistance, and insulin levels. It is also linked to lower blood pressure, blood rate, and blood pressure.

Ghrelin's positive effects include reduced inflammation and antiaging properties. It is also linked to slowing down cell-aging. Cell aging can lead to higher mortality and greater risks of developing diabetes. Obese people tend to have lower levels than normal of ghrelin. However, their reduction can lead to decreased benefits such as preventing cardiovascular disease and diabetes.

As you can see, both positive as well as negative effects can be had by ghrelin. This means that you can't reduce or eliminate ghrelin (or the feeling of hunger) when trying to balance hormones and eat healthier. Instead, you should retrain your brain and body to respond in a more controlled, balanced way. Ghrelin is more likely to be out of balance when your diet is unhealthy. This is especially true if you have sugar addictions or emotional eating. You will see positive changes in your weight and health if you eat mindfully.

How Weight Gain is Caused by Insulin Resistance and Hormonal Imbalance

I mentioned in the beginning that weight gain can be caused and maintained by many factors. Hormonal balance is one such factor. Hormonal imbalance is caused by poor diet, stress, sleep loss, poor nutrition, and chronic conditions such as cancer that are treated with strong medication. Hormonal imbalance either slows down metabolism, or causes blood glucose levels to be too high. If hormones are high, they can block or slowdown the absorption and cause blood glucose to become fat cells.

Here's how hormones impact weight gain (Pi Sunyer 2009.

* Thyroid. Hypothyroidism is also known as a slow thyroid. This condition can lead to weight gain. Your thyroid makes the hormones calcitonin (T3) and T4. Your pituitary gland excretes more TSH hormones when it produces less of these hormones. This hormone stimulates your thyroid, but it can also

slow your metabolism and heart rate and cause sluggishness.

* Leptin. Leptin, a hormone that signals satisfaction in a healthy person's body, is called. But, if you eat too many unhealthy food items, such as processed and sweet foods, your body may create additional fatty deposits, including in the liver and stomach. In this scenario, fat can also excrete leptin which can cause weight gain. This is when your brain stops responding to the signal that you should stop eating.

* Insulin. Insulin levels can rise due to increased consumption of processed foods or foods that are high in sugar. Insulin can build up in your blood and cause your cells to block it from entering. This causes insulin to become fat cells and feed them.

* Estrogen. Weight gain can also occur if estrogen levels are too high. Weight gain can also be caused by excessively

high or too low estrogen levels. When this hormone is too high it causes insulin resistance. If too low, it slows down the metabolism and makes all energy converted into fat.

* Cortisol regulates energy level and mobilization. If the levels are too high, they can lead to fat accumulation, leading to weight gain.

* A low level of progesterone is linked to weight gain and depression.

* Testosterone. Low testosterone levels, in both men as women, are associated with weight gains. Testosterone helps to reduce fat and strengthen bones and muscles. It is also known to cause an increased accumulation of fat if it is low.

* Melatonin. Your sleep cycle can be maintained with melatonin. You can have a decrease in the amount of this hormone produced by your pineal gland, or if you don't get enough rest, it

could cause a disruption to your sleep cycle. You can gain weight by being sleep deficient.

* Glucocorticoids. These hormones control how sugars, protein, and fats are used by your body. This hormone reduces sugar intake in the body after the body has healed from several periods of inflammation. The glucose that is not used up goes to fat cells.

Why Is Being Overweight Risky?

It can be frustrating to have to cope with weight gain, especially if your attempts to lose weight do not seem to be working. Because obesity can be due to many complex causes, it is not surprising that you won't see an immediate improvement in both your weight and overall health for several months or even years. It's better than doing nothing to improve your health and weight. You should learn more about weight gain and how it can lead to weight loss.

It is well-known that excess weight can lead to poor health. Obesity is associated to many diseases. We are studying the causes of obesity and the effects it has on your health.

What happens when you gain weight to your body?

* Hormonal imbalance. Increased weight can lead to changes in the hormone levels of your brain and body. This includes the chemicals in your brain. It can impact your health, mood, and overall well-being. Both the mental and physical effects of obesity (anxiety, depressive symptoms, heart disease, diabetes) share one thing in common: hormones. These chemicals affect how external sensations are perceived, as well as how your internal organs respond to foods.

* Anxiety and depression. It is common for one hormone or neurotransmitter to control many functions. This makes it difficult to understand the connections. One example of this is the brain's part that controls mood and forms habits. This creates a feeling for pleasure and reward in the form of healthy behavior. Being overweight affects the function of these areas which helps explain the link between obesity and depression.

Scientists have confirmed a link between physical health & mental state, but it remains to be determined how exactly this happens.

* Sleep problems. Increased weight is strongly related to sleep problems and correlates well with sleep apnea. Extra weight can make breathing more difficult and cause additional stress to your respiratory systems. With sleep apnea it is possible to temporarily stop breathing while asleep. This can lead to disturbed sleep. You may wake up often

and find it difficult to fall back asleep. This can cause further damage to your body and increase weight.

You should also remember that weight loss does not necessarily come from eating too many fatty meals. It's not so simple. Obesity is primarily due to an excess of fatty resources. But, fat gain doesn't always relate to food consumption. Hormonal imbalances may cause other substances (such as insulin) to travel into fat cells or build fatty tissues. Slow metabolism, caused either by hormonal imbalances and sleep deprivation as well as unhealthy lifestyles, can cause energy not to be expended but to be stored as extra fat. There is a condition called metabolic damage that can cause weight loss. When you eat too little or increase your physical activity, your mind may think and act as if starvation is imminent. Your metabolism slows to an extent. Although people claim they have lost weight, they still eat a lot after their weight loss programs are over. This is because metabolism focuses now on turning every bite of food into fat.

Perhaps the most grave link between obesity-related cancer is the one that exists. Researchers have found that excess weight can lead to 13 types cancers, accounting for nearly 40% of all cases (Centers for Disease Control and Prevention).

Although you won't get cancer if you are overweight, it will increase your chances. Bad eating habits, in addition to being linked with weight gain, increase the likelihood of getting cancer. The major problem is the impact of added sugars on the whole body, from the digestive system to the hormones.

* High blood Pressure High blood pressure and weight gain are linked with cardiovascular disease. You can

experience a dramatic increase in blood pressure if your heart is under strain from extra weight. High blood pressure correlates with dementia and stroke as well as diabetes.

* It is well-researched that obesity and diabetes can be linked. Nearly 90% diabetes patients are obese. As extra weight prevents the body's ability to use insulin as it normally would, (Poriese & al. 1995).

* Cholesterol (another blood chemical) is elevated in people who are obese. It can also be associated with high blood cholesterol and heart disease. Excess cholesterol in the blood can cause clogs, which can lead to serious health problems. High cholesterol is often caused by unhealthy eating habits, especially high-fat meals.

Unfortunately, there are times when excess weight can persist, regardless of your best efforts to maintain a healthy diet. A combination of low exercise and poor eating habits can cause weight gain. However, medications, hormonal imbalance, thyroid problems and other health issues can make it difficult for you to lose weight no matter what. For long-term results, it is important to get regular health checks and perform lab tests.

As I stated before, no matter what your success in losing weight, you should never stop praising yourself. Even if it seems like you are stuck in one area, you're not getting worse. That is progress. The bottom line is that you can avoid many unwanted consequences of weight loss by doing what you can to keep your body healthy.

* Increased food intake by losing your senses of taste

* Frequent migraines,

* High cholesterol

* Depression due to hormonal imbalance and poor body image

* Fertility problems that are caused by hormonal imbalances in adipose.

* Muscle pain from vitamin D deficiency. This is also associated with calcium deficiencies and chronic pains.

* Sleep Apnea and Snoring

* DNA modifications that lead to diabetes in both parents, and children

* Urinary issues can indicate kidney disease.

* Poor breathing and lack of good sleep

* * And other.

Chapter 3: Gastric Banding – A Last

Medical Resort

What is Gastric banding?

What if you try everything: diet, exercise, lifestyle change, etc., and still you are not losing weight. Sometimes, surgery can be required to facilitate the process. A surgeon will put a band around the stomach's top to perform laparoscopic gastroscopy. This will make it easier to eat smaller portions and create a small pouch for food. The band can even be adjusted after surgery. A surgeon can remove the band if needed to ensure that food moves more easily through your stomach. But how does this operation work?

What is Gastric Banding?

Gastric Banding is one option for those suffering from obesity. Bariatric surgery refers to surgeries that help with weight loss. Each of these procedures has its own unique characteristics, but they all result in a decrease in stomach size and consequently, a reduction of appetite. Bariatric surgery can result in smaller meals because you are fuller and feel fuller. Here's what gastric banding looks like:

Anesthesia will be used to anesthetize you. The general anesthesia is meant to make you completely unconscious and not feel any pain.

* The surgeon will then insert a camera into your belly. This is why laparoscopic surgery is so popular. The surgery uses very small incisions to access your inside and allows for greater insight.

* After this, the surgeon can make up five abdominal surgical cuts. These cuts will be very minimal, leaving you with

minimal scarring. These holes are used by the surgeon to navigate the camera or other instruments. The surgeon will insert a gastric band in your stomach without any additional cutting or stapling.

* This surgery is simple and quick, leaving you with minimal trauma. You'll find you can eat much more after surgery. The surgeon will make a small pouch in your stomach that fills quickly. It will slowly empty into your bigger stomach.

The insert is made with silicone, which has been approved and accepted by the Food and Drug Administration. It won't cause any injuries to your inner organs, or release any harmful toxins into your bloodstream.

In addition to placing the band, your surgeon will insert a tube under your abdominal wall. The doctor will inject saline through the tube to inflate your band after surgery. After your surgery is complete, the doctor will control the band's contraction to ensure that it performs well and you are comfortable. The goal of the surgery is to reduce food intake but not cause any discomfort.

This bariatric procedure will help you stop overeating, while still allowing for the appropriate amount of foods to be eaten. You won't be suffering from malnutrition which is common in calorie restriction diets.

This is minimally invasive surgery and you can go home the same day. No food is allowed after midnight, so you must prepare well. While you can return to your regular activities in just two days, it's best to take a week of leave to rest, recuperate and adapt to a new diet. It is important to understand how you feel about food and what meals you should eat during the day. It will take time to adjust.

Your diet should include only water and fluids following surgery. In the first days following surgery, lean soups or broths should be eaten. In the first 4 weeks after surgery, you should consume a variety of blended foods and pureed veggies. After the fourth weeks, you can start introducing foods. Six weeks after surgery, your normal diet may return.

There are restrictions on who can have this type of surgery. In the past, people with a lower BMI than 35 were eligible for this surgery. This applies to sleep apnea as well as high bloodpressure and diabetes. This means that surgery may be recommended if obesity-related complications pose a significant risk to your health.

However, technology advancements have made this surgery safer. If you have a BMI between 30 and 35, your physician may recommend surgery. First, your doctor may recommend you to increase your exercise and lifestyle, as well as taking medications to treat any health problems.

Most people aren't advised to have gastric bypass surgery if they have a history with drug or alcohol abuse, uncontrolled mental disease, or difficulty understanding the risks and benefits as well the lifestyle changes required.

What are the advantages of gastric banding

Gastric band surgery has many benefits. It increases the likelihood that you will lose weight over time. And, it is very quick to recover from. There are no complications following surgery. There is a small risk that you might get hernias, or other infections. This surgery can also reduce the risk of hypertension, diabetes, and incontinence. The surgery will result in a decreased stomach which won't lead to malnutrition. You will continue to be able consume and absorb the proper nutrients.

Patients frequently report a higher quality of life after the procedure. Your doctor has the ability to adjust your band and track your weight loss. A tightening of the band will decrease your appetite and reduce the size of your pouch. On the other hand, loosening can allow you to eat more.

People lose between 40-60% and 60% of their initial weight after having the gastric bands performed (Wittgrove & Clark (2000)).

What are the risks involved in gastric banding

While the risk is relatively low, this operation still has some risks. An allergic reaction to anesthesia can cause problems such as breathing, bloodclots or embolisms, or bleeding. You may notice a slower weight loss if you have other health conditions. The band can slip or may erode into your stomach. In such cases, the surgeon may need to remove the band.

15% of patients will require follow-up surgical treatment to resolve complications from a laproscopic gastric band. (Wittgrove & Clark 2001).

It is essential to strictly follow the diet recommendations given after the surgery. Overeating could cause vomiting or dilate your stomach.

Gastric band surgery is just like any other surgical procedure. It can injure your stomach, abdominal organs and intestines. There is also a possibility of gastrointestinal scarring. This can lead to bowel blockage and malnutrition.

Weight loss can be a good thing for your health, and it can even boost your confidence. Weight loss is not the only benefit of a gastricband. This surgery has the most long-lasting benefit. It can heal diet-related diseases as well as change the lifestyle and habits that caused overeating. Some people feel too hungry to resist eating even though it can be harmful to their overall health. It's easier to modify your eating habits when you have a reduced appetite.

People who are trying to reduce their weight and appetite have other options. Gastric bypass surgery is an option. This surgery involves applying staples to your stomach to reduce the size and attach it to your small intestine. This will not only reduce your appetite or food intake, but also affect your nutrient absorption. This surgery could also change the balance in your gut hormones. Additionally, it can be difficult to reverse the results.

Another option is to use the gastric Duodenal Switch. With this surgery, your doctor will direct the food into your smallintestine. Then, the surgeon will bypass the smallintestine. While this surgery leads to faster weight loss, there are higher chances of complications.

Another option would be to have a Sleeve Gastrectomy. This operation will remove more than half the stomach. This leaves a thin skin similar to a banana. As the stomach is removed, this procedure is irreversible. This procedure is becoming more popular because of its high success rates. There are also fewer complications. According to Wittgrove & Clark 2000, patients often lose 40-50% of their initial weight.

Sleeve gastrectomy could be performed by either a laparoscopically or through a surgically incision across the abdomen. The surgery can take four to six weeks to completely recover, similar to the gastric banding.

Mixed surgery is another option. This includes stomach stapling, which creates a small pouch. The pouch is then reconnected back to the smallintestine. The surgery does not result in a significant drop in food consumption but can reduce your nutrient intake.

This chapter has shown that gastric Banding is one of last resort options to reduce hunger. But what if surgery wasn't necessary? The next chapter will cover hypnosis as an option to increase your mental resources for changing your daily routine and losing weight.

Chapter 4: Hypnosis, Weight Loss And

Hypnosis

Research has shown that hypnosis is an effective tool for self improvement. The reason behind this simple conclusion is clear. Hypnosis reprograms your mind by changing your subconscious beliefs. Our subconscious beliefs are a major influence on our motivation, behaviors, assumptions, and decision-making (Holloway & Donald. You can change them from being negative to be positive, and you will see a positive shift in your relationship with food. The basis of a person's relationships with food are determined by their early childhood experiences. This relationship is further affected by how we handle challenges, stress, and difficult feelings as adults.

How Hypnosis is able to help you lose weight

Hypnosis can be described as a mental state that allows you to openly and readily accept suggestions. It is used to challenge unconscious patterns and help them change. Hypnosis can bypass the critical mind, allowing your mind to relax for long enough to open up to learning new things. By using hypnosis, many people are able to quit addictions, gain confidence, and increase self-esteem. This can be done by affirming positive beliefs, assumptions, and/or food related thoughts about yourself and the world.

If your mind is in this state of suggestibility and relaxation, it becomes easier to believe positive things. You might think that losing weight is possible and that exercise and physical activity are possible. Hypnosis can also bring back positive memories, experience, and associations which can help to shift your mindset.

Weight gain that is prolonged and continuous can cause people to lose confidence in their ability or capability to slim down. This belief leads to more unhealthy lifestyles, such as overeating or smoking. Hypnotherapy in this case helps you challenge negative assumptions regarding your competence. This is one key contributor to people who are able not only to lose weight but also to alleviate chronic pain and quit smoking or drinking through hypnosis.

When talking about thoughts, it is important to keep in mind that they can both be conscious and subconscious. Our minds can detect conscious thoughts, but the ones we don't have are far more powerful. They may even claim to rule from the shadows. They whisper quietly in our ears and create sudden sensations that cause fear, doubts or inadequacy. These thoughts arise from both early childhood experiences and adult experiences which could have been deeply painful and traumatic. Sometimes, they are too difficult to process.

Sometimes distress can be too intense to process and we tend to push it into the realms of the unconscious. This is applicable to difficult thoughts, feelings and memories. These things are not lost forever. Even worse, difficulties have a stronger impact on our behavior the harder we try.

Hypnosis assists in letting go of negative experiences and replacing self-scrutiny, with the ability to set and achieve empowering goals. This process must be extremely therapeutic and expert-led. You may find hundreds or thousands of weight loss audio hypnosis tracks online. But do they work? They're not made to help you overcome unconscious problems. If you could just affirm positive things to your self, it would make it much easier to reprogram yourself. But effective hypnosis centers around the individual's problems and guides them towards processing, letting go and then introducing affirmations.

How to Use Hypnosis To Lose Weight

You will be able to question and replace negative thoughts, experiences, and feelings related to weight loss and exercise with hypnosis. This will allow you to slowly shift your mindset.

The State Theory of Hypnosis claims that hypnosis is a way to alter your consciousness. This is a way to be able bypass conscious thoughts which alters normal brain processing. Another theory, the Non-state Theory of Hypnosis (Brown & Fromm 2013), suggests that people act like they're in hypnosis and change their behavior under the assumption they're being hypnotized. This is why people form beliefs about how they should behave after hypnosis.

Hypnosis allows us to perceive reality differently. Our perceptions are influenced significantly by our habitual patterns, according to studies (Horowitz (2006)). Hypnosis can effectively be used to improve the positive thinking patterns.

Our perceptions of reality are often distorted. This means that what we believe to exist doesn't necessarily have to be true. How our brain interprets the sensory information we receive can have a significant impact on how we perceive reality. This is called "top-down processing" and it means that the new data overrides the lower-level processes. Hypnosis is a process that gives you positive and helpful information. This helps to break bad habitual thinking.

It is essential to understand the root cause of the problem in order to make long-term improvements. First, examine the negative thoughts and their underpinning assumptions and then replace them with affirmative information. If your brain says you need sugar because you are upset, this is a top-down negativity. Hypnosis is a way to convince your brain that this is not true.

Reframe your preconditioned beliefs concerning food, weight, health, and body

Hypnosis can be used to override or reframe preconditioned beliefs. Preconditioned beliefs lead you to assign traits or attributes to objects and situations that do not have to be true. You might think that more expensive products equal better quality. Hypnosis can make you more susceptible to questioning your assumptions. Two distinct principles can be used when reframing thought pattern:

* Dissociation. Hypnosis allows one to examine whether a suggestion corresponds to existing thoughts and then gradually build new assumptions.

* Suggestion. You can focus on one idea when you hypnotise and you will be able to overlook your critical mind. Repeating this for a longer duration of time will allow you to train your brain to create or believe a different reality. You might find that the new perspective helps you avoid the mistaken belief that you have to smoke or eat when you're under stress.

According to Horowitz (2006), hypnotherapy can be used to treat the following conditions.

* Sleep disorders. Research has shown that hypnotherapy can increase slow-wave REM. It can actually increase REM sleep up to 80%.

* Weight gain. According to research, hypnosis helped people lose up 17 pounds.

* Smoking. Hypnotherapy was able to help smokers quit smoking. In fact, 82% of participants remained smokers six-months after the study.

* Addiction. * Addiction. More than 90% of people who received hypnotherapy remained drug-free for six consecutive months.

* Depression and anxiety. Long-term results of Hypnotherapy were highly successful in treating depression and anxiety.

Hypnosis Increases Confidence In Your Ability To Lose Weight

Along with physical, psychological, and environmental factors, weight-loss mindset has a huge impact. The main reason people have negative thoughts about weight loss is that they can't picture themselves being slimmer and healthier. While being overweight and managing health issues is difficult, it's the only reality many can accept. Hypnotherapy can help you to see and believe that you are capable of living a healthy, active, fit, strong, and happy life. Here are some ways that hypnotherapy aids in weight loss.

* Finding the root cause. Most therapists believe that our willpower and mind are the key to achieving whatever we desire. The majority of diet studies indicate that weight loss comes down to calorie reduction. However, long-term success and maintenance heavily depends upon diet satisfaction and nutrition richness. However, you may lose several hundred pounds in just a few short months. How does this impact your health? Do you think feeling unsatisfied after eating very little for the long-term sustainable? Most likely not. Many

scientists from different disciplines agree that long-term weight loss is possible by focusing on a balanced diet that works for you. There are many ways to feel satisfied, healthy, and enough about food. Many influences prevent you understanding the importance of eating and feeling satisfied.

* Positivity. You need to believe you can lose weight. Hypnosis helps to visualize and believe that you can eat healthier.

* See the good side. People can be either positively or negatively biased. Optimists often focus on the positives while underestimating real risks. However, pessimists focus only on the negatives. This makes it difficult for them to believe in positive things. Hypnotherapy gives you positive suggestions. You'll be able to see the value in hypnotherapy and how your body deserves love, respect,

compassion, and care. Your hypnotherapist helps you to identify your challenges and create your own mantras that you can use to overcome them.

* Visualization. Visualizing weight loss success can help you believe that your vision is possible. Hypnotherapy helps you to recall your feelings when you were healthier and leaner. It will also help you remember how you looked and feel. You can even visualize yourself in the future, putting yourself in the same position as your target weight. This reinforces your belief that you are capable of losing weight.

* Stop food cravings To reduce your appetite, imagine letting go all food cravings. Find other ways to entertain, celebrate, as well as to feel safe. As a result, you will start to lose weight.

* Additional treatment. Hypnosis is best used in conjunction with cognitive

behavior therapy. This allows you to challenge and question your negative self beliefs and underlying assumptions. CBT assists in the creation of realistic diets and exercise plans. CBT also looks at how to change your response to stressful situations so you don't overeat. Hypnotherapy helps you be more conscious of your thoughts by helping you to become more self-aware. It helps you relax and lets go of negative thoughts.

* Mental adjustment. It's difficult to break bad thought patterns. Also, positive thoughts will require constant work to reinforce and sustain. Hypnotherapy allows you to make small, but substantial changes when making spontaneous decisions, such as choosing to have a piece or fruit rather than chocolate.

* Increase your intuition. In the past, your instinctive responses were a problem in your efforts to lose fat and

become healthier. They can also be a friend and ally. Similar to the mechanisms that help you gain weight, our instinctive nature helps us recognize what we truly require, both emotionally and physically. Hypnotherapy enables you to transcend your learning patterns and tune in to your intuition. This helps you find your true needs. It will help you see that even though you might feel like you need pizza every night, you really crave friendship and connection. As you become more aware of your emotional needs, it will become easier to identify when your hunger is legitimate and when it's not.

* Repetition. Like other therapeutic methods, hypnotherapy can't make any noticeable changes right away. Your patience and persistence will be necessary, along with a gentle yet accepting attitude toward yourself. Accept that your present patterns took

years to build and cement. Changes in this manner are not only impossible, but potentially dangerous. You can't convince yourself into believing something you don't believe. Hypnosis helps to build up real-life proof of efficiency. You will see improvements over time, and you will become more confident in your abilities.

* Relapse management. You are human and you can fall back into old routines. Every relapse provides an opportunity for you to assess your belief system. Hypnotherapy aids in this process. Every time you "fail", it will be an opportunity for you to learn something about yourself and to show more love, acceptance, and compassion to yourself.

As you can see hypnotherapy is more about how you feel about your body and food. It also focuses on changing your eating habits. If you're still having trouble understanding hypnosis, you can think of it as the process of focusing and absorbing positive affirmations that are encouraging and motivating about yourself, your ability to lose weight, and others.

The hypnotherapist uses mental images and repetitions to do this. The experience is deeply relaxing and mentally rejuvenating. Hypnosis can be used to aid in weight loss and improve quality of your life. These are all essential conditions for long term weight loss. But, exercise is the only way to lose weight.

Hypnosis doesn't just remove insecurity about your ability to do things, but it also helps you resist cravings for food and avoid temptations. Weight loss is possible by maintaining a long-term plan and exercising when you feel like it. A positive, encouraging mindset can make it much easier.

Many people who have seen success with hypnotherapy for weight loss say that it takes time. The mindset shifts slowly and steadily. At first you may notice it becoming easier to stop eating when your stomach is full. This is vital because losing weight can be difficult if you are unable to identify when you've had enough. You may still eat regularly for emotional reasons or with friends but you will have less urge to finish the meal.

You might find that you have a more conscious relationship with food. The loss of taste is a sign of obesity. After regular hypnosis, it might be that you have a greater appreciation for food flavors and textures. This subjective feeling of satisfaction can increase, meaning it will make you eat less. Additionally, better food experiences can bring more pleasure from fewer foods. By taking your time, learning to taste food and taking the time to enjoy it, you will be able eat slower and more easily find satisfaction and satisfaction from smaller portions.

Over time you'll develop the willpower to eat according a program that is reasonably healthy for you. This will make it easier to maintain a healthy diet. It will no longer be difficult to cook often or to carefully choose the right groceries for you when grocery shopping. You will be able to have patience and become more self-aware about food and eating. Gradually you'll learn to not only understand the instinctive desires of your body, but also how they came about. For example, you might discover that a sugar craving is not caused by true hunger but an imbalance in your body. This will make it easier for you to resist. Or you might be able to recognize that you are about to prepare a meal just to occupy your mind. With this understanding, you may decide to go on a walk or read.

Hypnosis for Weight Loss aims to support you in developing healthy eating habits. It will change your perception of food, and allow you to approach food in a more relaxed, calm way. In addition to understanding your appetite, you'll also feel more motivated, as you will have an intuitive sense of what you should eat. The best benefit of hypnosis is in the ability to understand your relationship to food and draw associations with emotions. The journey to weight loss will be easier if you can do that. In addition, you'll find new ways to handle difficult situations. This will add another mental benefit to your overall well-being and quality of living.

Hypnosis should, when done well, feel comfortable and relaxed. You should relax but not fall asleep. Your attention must be focused inwards. Hypnosis feels nothing like a deep trance. You will always be in control and awake. Many people find the idea hypnotized can make them feel frightened. As you can see, hypnosis slowly over a long duration of time leads to changes that are good for your health. Hypnotized people still have the ability to exercise their willpower and make decisions.

However, hypnosis is not without its limitations. If it's done at the therapists office, it can cost quite a bit for a treatment that requires many repeats in order to achieve results. The cost of the treatment is usually increased. You pay to have time with a licensed professional who is skilled in helping you to identify the causes and to find the authentic, real, and authentic ways to overcome these obstacles. Even so, investing thousands of bucks in a therapy that doesn't immediately produce improvement can cause some to doubt. It is possible to permanently change the way you think by changing your mind.

Hypnosis does have another advantage, even though the wait time can seem frustrating. It is essential to address all health issues before you can use hypnosis. Hypnosis encompasses all the changes made through exercise, dieting, and medical treatment. This is not a claim that it can make weight loss happen by itself. A major motivation booster is also the knowledge gained through hypnosis about the importance of receiving treatment for other health conditions. You can show your competence in losing weight by doing every little thing that you can to improve your health. This will improve your self-image and confidence, as well as motivate you to take an active approach to healing and recovery from obesity related diseases.

Hypnosis for weight loss has many benefits, but not all people are able to take the helpful suggestions. Research suggests that some people have brains that aren't able to take in suggestions. People who don't have the ability to think creatively or are not very imaginative are called those. If you are more down-to earth and have difficulty with imagination, it is possible that you will need to make an effort to listen to hypnotherapists or record hypnosis.

It is possible to compare hypnosis to a feeling like you are sleeping but in a concentrated manner. Being in a state or suggestibility allows you to be guided toward different visualizations and thoughts. Hypnosis is a technique that involves you looking at a display or board to see an image of what is being suggested. This will allow you to experience things that you aren't experiencing in your current life and help you accept them.

It's important to know that a hypnotic mental state is not something you suddenly experience or that you do. It's a mental state that usually occurs throughout the day. You can only trigger and enter hypnosis willingly and purposefully. There are many ways to induce the hypnototic state of mind. The first method is to simulate falling asleep. This will induce a mental state between being awake, and being asleep. This opens up certain areas of your brain and removes some barriers. Guided visualizations will place you in different environments. You can use guided visualizations to help you visualize different environments and situations.

Your therapist may also make unrelated statements that you don't understand or find confusing. This is done to prevent you from falling asleep. This encourages deep healing by allowing for more relaxation.

Chapter 5: Gastric Band Hypnosis

Welcome to gastric band-hypnosis. This hypnosis will help to lose weight, but you don't have to go under the knife. The therapy's first component will be to identify the root cause of emotional eating. You will recall all negative experiences that you might have had with food. Next, identify and admit to any unhealthy eating habits. After that, you will have a visualized gastric band surgeon. This will make it possible to visualize a gastric bypass.

Part One

Your body will start to recognize the messages and respond in a way that lessens your appetite. Like the gastric bands, you will find yourself feeling fuller with smaller meals. As you imagine going through this procedure, the more you do it, the better your body's response to the suggestions. You will feel your stomach shrink and you will have more energy to satisfy your desires. The procedure will look and feel more real with each repeat, and you will experience a more tangible effect.

First, let us briefly discuss diets. Next, let us address the reasons why you may not have been able to lose weight in past years. Failing to follow through with a diet wasn't your fault. Allow yourself to feel the shame and guilt associated with trying to maintain a steady diet in the recent past. Most diets are temporary in nature and difficult to sustain for the long-term. It isn't you who are the problem. Your problems with dieting were caused by the fact that restrictive diets don't work. They do not just restrict food and nutrients, but also provide the satisfaction and pleasure that is necessary for long-term success.

The hypnosis can help you make a conscious commitment to your own eating habits. As you subconsciously receive the virtual band around your stomach, you'll gradually, through suggestions and confidence, learn the skills necessary to make healthy eating choices. These habits will have a direct impact on how you eat, move through your day, exercise, etc. The beneficial changes will continue to build over time and support long-term, healthy weight reduction, as well as improving your physical fitness.

Let's talk about your weight loss and eating habits. Next, we will discuss your relationship with food and your general health.

Recall what you experienced with previous treatments, as well as the reasons for your failure. It's possible to recreate the experience of gastric band operation by re-creating it. The entire procedure will be carried out in a deep hypnotic sleep state. This hypnosis will guide your through the procedure step by step.

To begin hypnosis, imagine yourself going into anesthesia and relaxing. After that you will be taken through the process to have your gastric band fitted, from the first cut, all the way to the final fitting. You can even get hypnotized through the process of sewing your cuts.

While the process unfolds in front of you, you'll also be guided to feel the sights and sounds around. This will help you feel more connected to the world and make it more real. You will slowly convince your subconscious mind that the experiences you have are real.

In addition to simulating surgery, the hypnosis program will offer suggestions to boost your self-confidence. You will be provided with additional methods to practice at your home after the procedure.

Part Two

Welcome to your gastric hypnosis. The hypnosis will provide you with a virtual graph of your gastric band. You can lose weight naturally and in a healthy manner for your mind, body, and soul. Remember that your mind is always in control. These suggestions will benefit you and are helpful and positive. This hypnosis can be repeated whenever you want.

First, let us relax and allow our minds to be open to positive suggestions. Your mind should be able to relax and become more positive. You'll begin to receive suggestions for relaxation so that you can mentally and literally install the Hypnotic Gastric Band.

Relax. Focus on my voice. As you listen more to my voice, your relaxation increases. Keep relaxing, shrugging, and dropping your shoulders to release any tension. To identify any discomfort or tightness, look around. If tension is detected, you can relax the tight area. Relax all areas that you feel unwell.

I will now count down from ten, to one. After I finish counting you will feel completely relaxed. All parts of your body will feel fully relaxed.

* Ten. Breathe in. Take a moment to pause. Next, let the breath go. Relax and take a deep inhale.

* Nine. Then, take a second pause and let the breath out.

* Eight. * Eight. You now feel so much better.

* Seven. * Seven. Inhaling in relaxation means that you are also breathing out tension, discomfort, and stress. With

each breath, you become calm and peaceful in your mind.

* Six. You become calmer and more peaceful. Everything around is calm, peaceful, and safe. You can only hear this hypnosis. All worries, chores, stress, and other concerns fade away.

* Five. You're only focusing on my voice. Breathe out tension and relax. Every exhale brings you deeper into relaxation. Deeper, deeper, until you feel totally safe and light.

* Four. Relaxation ishes across your face, jaw, and your lips. Your neck is softening, your shoulders are relaxed. Relaxation flows throughout your body. This includes your shoulders and back, your chest, stomach, and chest. You are softening and easing your thighs, calves, as well as your feet. You feel comfortable, safe, and relaxed. As you take deep inhale and exhale, your relaxation is deeper.

Your hands are at your side, fully relaxed. There is no need for you to move. All that matters is that your mind and body are calm and relaxed. Relaxing further is the only way to go. Your body is opening up and softening.

As you exhale your body sinks further into the chair. Letting go feels beautiful. You are floating through heavy relaxation.

* Three: Your legs feel heavier. As your feet become looser and calmer, you will be able to concentrate on your feet.

* Relaxed at two. Remember, you are in charge.

* One. You are letting yourself go of all that is not necessary for relaxation. You are relaxed, at ease, and totally comfortable. You are relaxed and comfortable, and your mind is open. You are open to receiving my suggestions. Your mind, body, and spirit are interconnected. You can open your

mind right now. To improve your abilities and resources, you must accept positive, constructive ideas. Your mind is clear. You look forward the change you see coming.

You feel happy and calm. This positive change will make your life more enjoyable, vibrant, and full of energy. You are positive and excited about a positive outcome.

You are in a hospital corridor. You can hear and see visitors. You can smell the disinfectants and clean hygiene products. Everything is fresh and clean. You are in control and you're about to change how you view food. You are making positive changes in your body and mind.

A hospital bed is where you are currently lying. A nurse is standing beside you. She is here to help. She is supportive and calm. The nurse smiles at me. You trust the nurse and feel like you can smile back at it. You feel comforted and happy when she touches you. The bright lights are everywhere.

Bright blue and white lights surround you. These lights make your sleepy and tired. Your eyes feel heavy while your breath is fresh and light.

There are many others there, and you feel as if you're sinking deeper and deeper into anesthesia.

It is a feeling that your stomach experiences. The excitement and safety of a fresh start are the most important things. You will feel comfortable in this space, surrounded with warm blue lights.

Be at ease in the hospital bed's softness. You should feel comfortable and relaxed as the bed supports you back. The nurse points a brightly lit light at you and you can only make out the shadows from medical staff. The nurse points a bright light at you, and you can only relax and take in the experience.

A cold sensation touches your stomach. Something inside starts to change. Your mind drifts away and you begin to observe yourself lying on the bed. You start to see doctors, nurses, instruments around you. Now, a doctor makes an incision in your stomach. They then attach the band to your stomach. It is fast over.

Now you can see that the staff has left. Everyone is happy and content, and so are we. The job has been completed. That was enough. You are becoming better each day. Your thoughts about food can be completely controlled by your mind.

Now, you are free to choose to eat wisely and to only consume the best food. These foods nourish your body and mind. You only want nutritious, high-quality meals.

The sensation of eating food is wonderful. They are nutritious, delicious and satiating. You only want healthy, lean, nourishing food in the ideal amounts. Your stomach feels comfortable and light. This is what your subconscious, conscious and subconscious minds decide. You feel at home. You feel calm, energized and hydrated. You deserve to feel strong. You have everything you require to get the fittest, healthiest body possible. As you eat the right amount, you will notice a difference in how full your stomach feels. Your stomach doesn't feel full anymore.

You now have healthy eating habits and a healthy attitude about food. You are now looking forward to being healthier and more in tune with your body. Everything works just as it should. You eat only when your stomach is full. It is possible to feel the difference in sadness and hunger as well as fear and hunger. Deep inhale, deep exhale these emotions. Take a few deep breathes and let it go. You don't have to cover them with food. You can relax and let your mind drift off.

As you breathe, you are constantly changing. Each breath brings you closer to your goals. You are confident in who you are. You view yourself in many different ways. You believe that you have the ability to make positive changes in your daily habits.

How you think and behave will be affected by how you feel. You are choosing to properly eat. You're choosing not to eat when you don't feel hungry. Within weeks, you will see changes as your body and brain learn to listen. This is the effect that hypnoband can have on your body and mind. You feel more in control. You feel right. You eat right. Your stomach is flat. You have a calm and positive attitude. You don't desire overeating. After a few weeks, you start to feel more energy. You see more possibilities and opportunities when you are calm and clear.

You feel proud about your achievement and you smile. You try on new clothes and find it easy to fit in them. You're more energetic and excited.

You enjoy being active and moving. You like healthy food, as well as the softness and flavour of protein, fruits,, and vegetables. You grow stronger and are slimmer. Your posture is more upright, with your head up. Friends, family, or colleagues notice how much you look healthier and how much more energy you have. Everything is right where it should be. You are healthy, happy, and in control.

Your belief system will remain intact as you allow the body and mind to enjoy healthy, nutritious foods in all their necessary quantities. Do not try to get to sleep. If you want to get up in the morning, you will be energized. You are looking forward for your day. Now, I will count between one and three. One, the energy has returned to your body. It is from your feet down to your head. You are now fully present and aware to the energy that is flowing through your body. Three, you're opening your eyes. You're alert and aware that something extraordinary has occurred.

After the Hypnosis

After going through the entire process of gastric bands hypnosis, your body will start to crave healthier foods. The subconscious suggestions that you were given will help your brain send the message to your brain that you are full even if you eat less. If you overeat, you'll start to notice that you're physically full. This might have been difficult in the old days. The difference between hunger and fullness will be easier to see with hypnosis. You'll notice tiny, barely detectable physical sensations when hungry. Also, you'll start to notice how you feel after eating. This will provide the foundation for healthy eating habits.

You will also feel more at ease and relaxed while hypnotizing.

Gastric band hypnosis allows you to reap the full benefits of the treatment, while avoiding the physical side effects of recovery. There won't be any nausea, acid reflux, or vomiting. You won't feel any symptoms from the surgery as it is entirely psychological. It depends on many factors whether or not gastric bandhypnosis works for you. Some people notice changes in behavior or sensations right away, while others may need to go back several times before they notice significant changes. You need to be patient and allow your mind and body to change in a natural way.

Trusting the process, feeling relaxed, and enjoying it are key factors for best results. You'll be able to make progress faster if you hold on to the positive beliefs. It will help put your mind at ease and allow you calmly to feel and sense the core issues.

Relaxation on a subconscious or cognitive level will help open your mind to positive suggestions. On a hypnotic, relaxation will enable you to relax and allow you to see the possibilities. You can release some negative beliefs through the simple act if reasoning. Most likely, you will be able to let go of some of your subconscious beliefs once you realize that they're not true.

Chapter 6: Complimentary Hypnosis

Using A Wholistic Approach

Hypnosis in Binge-Eating

The hypnosis page will help you to overcome binge-eating. Binge eating is when you can't cope with your true feelings. This hypnosis will help you get rid of your suppressed feelings and learn how to process them in a healthy, balanced way.

Slowly and evenly count from 10 up to 1. Ten. Ten. Nine. Calm down and allow your thoughts and feelings to flow. Do not try to change them or suppress them. Some of these thoughts, feelings and thoughts might surprise or make you feel uncomfortable. Eight. Ten. Seven. Focus on accepting your feelings and affirming that all your emotions are positive. They exist because they are important. Six. Accept them.

Five. On multiple levels, it is helpful to learn to accept and embrace your feelings. You will notice a decrease in overeating. Your barriers to feeling the best you can are being removed. Four. This will help you notice when your stomach starts to churn with emotions such as stress, fear and shame. Three. The ability to feel these feelings can help you have more control over your decision making. Two. Breathe in, out, and relax your entire system. One. Imagine yourself drifting into complete relaxation.

Now, work on revealing any emotions you might be suppressing. Accept that you now have the right to feel your feelings. Respond to them in the same way as you would any other person.

Your anxiety should be your focus. You will no longer be anxious if you are feeling stressed.

If you feel depressed, you'll be able to recognize the feeling and acknowledge it. Depressed feelings will make it clear that you need more action to solve your problems. If you're feeling frustrated, it's time to change your attitude towards the problem. Stress means you have to take it slow and complete as much work as you can.

You feel lonely when you don't have any human contact. Instead of eating, it is better to talk to someone. Perhaps you will volunteer or join an organization that revolves around you interests.

It is now that you understand that eating doesn't satisfy your feelings. These feelings will return. Now, listen to what your feelings are telling you. Listen to your feelings. Also, you'll notice the associations between certain emotions and overeating situations.

Hypnosis and Emotional Eating

This is the hypnosis for emotional eating. Relax your entire body by laying back. Relax your muscles beginning at your tip, up to your neck, shoulders, head, neck and shoulders, then moving down to your stomach and hips, thighs and calves. You can take the following few minutes and be yourself. If you have any troubled thoughts, accept them gently and let them go.

Now take a few deep inhalations. Close your eyes. Breathe slowly. Imagine floating on the peaceful ocean surface as waves wash away tension, stress, and other negative emotions. Think about the gentle rocking sound, the ocean's smell, and the sounds from the waves and seagulls that transport you into relaxation. Let's start counting down from 10 to 1. Picture white numbers in front your eyes. These numbers could be 10, 9, 8, 7, 6, 5, 6, 5, 4, 3, 3, 2, and 1. Now, relax.

This is the time to start to think about your relationship and food. Think back to your childhood. What was the most memorable memory of food? It may be with your entire family, or it could be just you. What is your feeling? What do you feel? Are you satisfied and happy? Or maybe you feel ashamed or tense. Spend some time examining your past.

Let's now go into your teens, and then into your adult life. What are you most fondly able to recall? Do you remember feeling anxious or nervous at times? Are there any memories of eating to seek consolation or relief? If so, bring back those memories. Examine how you felt.

Then ask yourself why do you feel hungry when trying emotions arise. Do you feel like you are trying to keep away from trauma, stress, sadness, or other negative emotions? Perhaps you eat when it makes you feel afraid. Accept that you made the decision to let your true feelings out. Now, acknowledge any difficult feelings.

Maybe you believed feeling angry, sad or scared made your weak. You might remember being shamed for feeling down or in need of support. If you have any memories of such times, it is important to remember them and give yourself the support, love and consolation that you deserve. You're now making a decision to love and respect your feelings. It is your choice to respond to them with compassion, acceptance and understanding. These feelings are not a sign of weakness or inadequacy. You also don't fear being wronged and becoming irresponsible. You are a strong, mature and responsible adult who takes full responsibility for your actions. You are fully capable of responding appropriately to any distress you may feel.

Now, make a vow to yourself to get better at processing your emotions. Take a moment to think about the last time this happened. Are there any emotions that you associate with this moment? Are you embarrassed? Do you feel incompetent? Let these emotions flow through your body. Give yourself permission to feel these emotions. Be compassionate for how you feel right now.

Pay attention when you are feeling in distress to your physical sensations. Do you feel your heart beating faster? Do you feel any tension? Are your limbs stiff? Are your fists tightened and clenched? If so, release your tension. Deepen your breathing and declare that you are accepting of the way you currently feel. Breathe out, and tell yourself that you're choosing not to feel these difficult emotions. You're choosing not to judge yourself and allow yourself to feel what you feel next time you're feeling in distress. Promise yourself that you won't suppress your emotions.

Now let's take a trip to a more peaceful place. Remember a time when your self-esteem was high. This feeling? Were you proud of your achievements? Perhaps you felt a sense of warmth and a smile on your face. Remember a time when your self-confidence was high and you were happy with yourself. What did you think of yourself in this scenario? Did you feel proud or humbled by the way you handled the situation? Did you feel smart or competent? What lessons have you taken away from this experience

This positive experience is what you choose to remember the next time that you feel down. You are choosing the memories of times when you felt proud, confident, creative and competent. When you have a hard feeling, you'll give yourself the love you deserve. Instead of denying your feelings, you will choose to think about the meaning of them. Instead of eating you will go for a walk, or talk to a friend. Do your best to inspire compassion, love, happiness, and joy in others. Be proud of yourself. When you take in, be proud of yourself for honoring your feelings. When you breathe out, acknowledge your decision to improve your face and process feelings.

Now you are returning to awareness. Now you are fully aware and alert to your surroundings. Be gentle with your eyes. Spend some time pondering your experience. Then, bring that feeling of satisfaction and fulfillment into every day.

Hypnosis and Cultural Eating

Let's get started on the hypnosis. First, find a quiet, comfortable space. The space should make you feel comfortable. It's best to be alone in a peaceful area, away from distractions. Perhaps your favorite chair will allow you to relax. If you have a TV, cellphone or other distractions, turn them off. If you live in a relationship with another person, let them be aware that you want to be by yourself and shouldn't be disturbed.

Let's get ready now to enter the hypnosis state. In hypnosis you will not fall asleep. You can rest assured that you are aware and in control your mind, body and emotions. Hypnosis is a way to make sure you do not do something you don't like.

Consider why you want hypnotized. What are your goals when you use hypnosis for this purpose? What is it you want to achieve with hypnosis. While focusing on the goal, relax. Relax and let the mind wander. You may be familiar with the way hypnosis feels if you've tried it before. Perhaps you are familiar with how it feels for you to receive suggestions. If so, you shouldn't place any expectations upon yourself.

You should pay attention to the tone, voice and overall vibe of this session. Find a place to relax and calm yourself, physically or mentally. Breathe deeply, evenly, and naturally. Let my words gently sweep over your head and shoulders. Remember that you're safe. You are calm, peaceful, and secure. You are in complete control of your body and mind.

It is important to remember that only suggestions that can benefit your body, mind and soul will be accepted. Acceptance of suggestions is only a decision you make.

Now, just focus on your breathe. Inhale and exhale slowly and evenly. Your lungs will fill up as you breathe in. When you exhale, let your body release any remaining tension, pressure, or dissatisfaction. Now, keep your focus on one point. It could be anywhere within the room, or any small object you choose. You can close your eyes, and just focus on the area between your eyebrows.

Now, relax each section of your body. To begin, concentrate on the top portion of your head. Let go of any feelings of stress. Next, you can focus on the top of your head, your eyes, your eyebrows, your jaw, your mouth, your mouth, and your cheeks. Relax your jaw, so it's not too tight. But not too much that it opens your mouth. To loosen tension in your neck, you can still relax your head and keep your head straight. Do the same with your shoulders. You can focus your attention on your chest. Now relax any tension in that area. Then you can move on to your stomach.

Allow all muscles to relax and become lighter, starting from your head down to your feet. Allow the waves and relaxation to flow over you. As you breathe in, let them fall. Relax and let these waves carry you into relaxation.

When you're listening to these words, pay attention to my voice. As you are gently floating into relaxation focus on my voice. This will help you to go deeper and deeper into an ever-growing state of softness and safety. You are sinking deeper into relaxation. You feel more relaxed the deeper you relax.

You have now found a place that is safe, enjoyable, and liberating. Perhaps it's a field or a beach. A staircase is visible as you gaze down. You will feel calmer and less anxious as you fall. Finally, you have reached the top of the staircase. Now, you see a small door in front. By opening the door, you enter a place of pure relaxation.

You are seeing yourself as a young child. Your family is around you. You might be in the kitchen or in a diner. The symbols of your culture will be displayed on the walls. What are those symbols you ask? What does that symbol represent to you? Look at the items on the table. Which foods are at the table? How do you feel about these food choices? Do these foods make you feel hungry? Or, are you satiated? How does the world react when you grab a bite to eat? Are they happy or judgemental? How will they respond if you decline to give them food? Is it offending? Are they dissatisfied?

Often, we eat to please our friends and family. We eat to make others happy or be part of a celebration. What if you don't want to eat on these occasions. As an adult, picture yourself in this space. Now, look at what is in front of your face. Consider this a safe space. You won't be judged if you eat or refuse to eat.

How do your feelings change? Get a bite if your stomach is feeling full. You can also enjoy the joy by not eating. Now you realize that you have the option to choose. Food doesn't impact your relationships with family or friends. Imagine yourself having fun talking, laughing, or even eating.

Are you beginning to feel hungry even if it wasn't previously? If so, think about why. What thoughts and feelings are you having that lead to this hunger?

Think of something funny to say to people who want to eat together. Instead of reaching down for a bite of food, imagine talking with the person you love. Allow yourself to feel joy and share intimacy with your loved-one.

You are now aware that eating is not necessary to bond.

Why do you eat? Are you trying avoid awkward questions or are you really trying to avoid them? Are there unresolved conflictual issues you wish to distract from? If so then you need to look at the person who causes your emotions. Tell them how you feel about their behavior. Tell them that you feel ashamed, hurt and sad about what they are asking. Tell them you're free to enjoy their company, and that you don't have to answer any awkward or embarrassing questions. Accept that you are entitled to feel the way it feels, but instead eat, feel safe and secure. You can let go any stress by exhaling and focusing your attention on the conversations and laughter at dinner. Begin to notice how your appetite improves.

Now imagine everyone leaving this room. You are the only one. The room is flooded with morning light. It's morning and you're about to get started. Your stomach is empty. It's time you connect with your intuitive side and learn how your meals are measured.

Imagine that a table in front you is filled with different foods. With an empty plate in hand, you now have to begin to examine the food. What foods does your body love? What are the best foods for your body and mind that are healthy? Grab your empty plate and begin to reach for the food. You will be able to observe how you arrange the fruits, vegetables, proteins, or dairy. What amount do you need for your stomach? Pay attention. First, you might reach to grab any food that looks delicious. Your full plate. How full is your plate?

Maybe your plate is overflowing with food. Consider removing foods from your plate if this is the case. Are there any foods you don't like or that are just too fat? If so, place them back into their bowls and don't feel embarrassed. This should be done slowly, each one at a while, acknowledging that it is your right to not consume foods you feel deprived of. This will give you the perfect portion size. Pay attention to what is on your plate. What's in your plate? What have you eaten?

Think of how you would feel if you felt hungry. Imagine you taking one bite at once, while enjoying the delicious food. Soon, your stomach is full. No longer do you need to eat. It's time for you to stop. Leave any remaining food on your table. Get up and go. Now, look at the food on your plate. You don't even have to eat all of your meal.

Only eat enough food to feel satisfied. You'll be satisfied when you feel you have eaten enough. You won't feel shame or guilt. You will now be able to eat as much or as little as you wish. It is your right choose only healthy foods. Be aware of the sensations of satiation and pleasure in you stomach. Your stomach feels full but not too full. Breathe in and experience the pleasure of knowing the nutrients from your fruits, vegetables and meats have now been converted into energy within your body. You can feel the energy flowing from your stomach into you muscles, bloodstream, brain. Consider the health foods that fuel your body and keep it healthy and strong. Now is the time to focus on your feelings of pride and pleasure.

Look around the room until you find a way to get out. This is where you will find the door that will allow you to regain your full awareness. Then, walk to the door. Take another deep breath, and that feeling of well-being, joy, and satisfaction will last for a while. Now, your stomach can communicate with you and tell you what foods to eat. As you exhale out, walk through the door. Pay attention to the sensation in your stomach. Keep in mind that each day you are reconnecting with your true self. You're also improving your intuition to choose what, when and how many meals you'll eat. You now know that you don't need to eat to be involved in your cultural and/or social activities. Bring this knowledge to every day.

Motivation to Workout Using Hypnosis

This hypnosis will make you more eager to work out. Exercise is important, and it's good for you. Yet, there is a part in you that doesn't want exercise. Waiting for the right time and the right place or company to do it is a common problem. Although it might seem difficult, exercising can be easy. With determination and drive, you'll find the motivation to exercise regularly.

By using positive suggestions and Hypnosis, you can create the desire and motivation for exercise and make it a regular part of your day. All you have to do is relax. Relax and close your eyelids. To focus inward, let go of any tension or stress. Keep your eyes on your intention to exercise with joy and pleasure. Notice how relaxed your body feels. Breathe in. Inhale relaxation. Allow stress to go as you let out.

Hypnosis can slow down time. Your mind is free to create the world of possibilities. There are no limitations. All you need to make your dreams come true is imagination. You are aware and present with thoughts, feelings, emotions, and sensations. You are opening up more to your inner world, becoming more aware. You are completely in control. You drift as you breathe. Imagine you are outside, enjoying the freshness of the air. It could be night or day, depending on your comfort level. You feel secure and protected.

You start to see a huge bonfire in front. As you draw closer, you begin to feel the warmth and energy surrounding your body. You feel warm and relaxed. It replenishes you with healing energy that will restore your entire being. This warm energy flows throughout the body. Your muscles are relaxes and letting go. Your entire body is relaxing, starting at your feet and ending at your head. Warm energy fills and relaxes the muscles. It softens your forehead, neck, & head. Gazing into the flame is a way to relax and let it go.

These flames contain your love and creative drive. They represent your inner strength.

Inhale and inhale this warmth. It will expand and grow. You breathe in healing energy, passion, and love. When you exhale, your body releases energy and passion that fuels growth. From three to one. With every breath, the fire gets stronger. With each breath, the fire grows deeper. Your mind opens to the warmth and influence these passions have on you, to the dreams that become a reality.

Two, it is easier to be relaxed. You are being more open to your imagination and eager to discover your passion. One. You are ready plant the seeds of drive and passion in your mind. Your mind is open and willing to listen to positive ideas. You know everything you want is best for your interests. These suggestions will be your reality if you are willing to accept them.

You love to exercise. You know exercise is good. You know you have the desire and passion to exercise each day.

You recognize that you need to let go all your fears and excuses to rediscover your passion. You can look into the fires of your passion, and choose to let go insecurity. Take a deep breath and let go of the insecurity. Look down. Below, you will find sticks and stones to represent your thoughts, fears, doubts, and pains related to movement, exercise or your physical capabilities and body.

Then, take the pieces you have collected and put them in the fire. Toss each piece one at a.m., and watch as they turn to ash. They become ashes, and all of your troubles, fears, and resentments will vanish. They fuel your drive to succeed.

All your fears melt away as the items are tossed into the fire. As they vanish, you can feel your need to exercise. Keep an eye on each one and try to understand their meanings. When you're done, say goodbye. Watch your love, motivation, or desire for growth, as they burn all around the fire. Keep searching for more obstacles, and keep throwing them into your fire. Focus on the passion and love within, and let them go. Now, notice the little seed. It inspires you to exercise. Plant it somewhere you love and it will grow.

Look around for a suitable spot to plant your garden. Pick a location that represents joy, peace of mind, love, and passion. Anywhere you choose is ideal. Plant the seed, firmly planting it in your mind. Now you will experience joy, happiness and love every time you exercise. This place grows stronger and more every time you exercise. It is essential to nourish this seed by working out. Your drive grows stronger with every day you exercise.

Take a look at yourself in two weeks. Your seed is now fully grown. Your seed is stronger, leaner and more driven. Your seed blooms. In a few years, you will see the results. Your seed has turned into a beautiful, healthy garden. It is a sacred place of joy. You can think about how you planted the seed and grew it through motivation and exercise. This garden produces fruits that you can only harvest. They keep your body and mind healthy. These fruits will keep your body young and beautiful. The sky is your view. See yourself working out. Notice the exercise. What are you doing with which of the following exercises? What changes is your body making as you exercise? How has your wellbeing and health improved? Be proud of the changes you've made. What were those changes? How can exercise improve your body, mind, spirit, and drive?

Consider yourself smiling and learning. You are exercising consistently and frequently and it feels great. It's therapeutic and refreshing. Your garden is always growing and producing fruit every time you exercise. These fruits can fuel your health, vitality and beauty.

Now, bring your attention back to the now. These memories can be kept with you, and taken into the new day. Changes are now possible. It is clear that you have established new beliefs and habits in your head. Every day you feel more motivated and committed. Exercise is a way to harvest the fruits that you have planted. Your passion grows, and it feels rewarding.

You can count from three to one. As you count, you will either fall asleep or wake up to become alert. You'll feel motivated, determined, and dedicated the next day you open your eyes. These changes now influence your reality.

Hypnosis for mental strength and willpower

This hypnosis will help increase your mental strength and willpower. Relaxe and take a deep breath. Close your eyes. You can relax all your muscles by scanning your body. You'll notice increased tension where you feel the muscles relax. Relax these areas, and let go of any tension. You are also becoming more relaxed from the inside, as your muscles relax. You breathe deeply, evenly, and softly.

You feel completely relaxed. You feel relaxed inside. You will notice how the relaxation spreads from your head to your shoulders and stomach to your legs to your toes.

Keep your eyes on your chest. You are breathing easy, and relaxing with each breathe. Outside sounds don't matter. Relaxation will spread through your body. You are completely aware, conscious, & in control. All your stomach muscles are relaxing down to the feet, knees or ankles. It feels good to feel calm, relaxed, and calm. For a second, take a deep breath and count down. As you count down, more relaxation ishes over you.

Five, you are letting loose of tension. Four, relax your body. You are exhaling here. You're now inhaling again.

Your success will bring you rewards. Your success hinges on what you do. It is common to want to finish the work you have started. Go for a walk or stick to a weight loss plan. You may have a strong urge to eat, intense feelings, or boredom.

This hypnosis can help you get rid of boredom. Perhaps you feel like your goal is to be successful but aren't sure how to do it. Sometimes, you lose sight of the goal. It makes one feel horrible. You'll have memories of the times you gave up and the opportunities missed.

You should pay attention to the spaces where these memories take place. How does this space look? How does it feel? How do you feel during these events?

How does it feel to feel bored and ready give up? How does it feel to quit

128

your diet after just a few days? How does it feel missing another workout?

Do you ever feel sad? What is it like to give in? How does it affect your life? Does it make you feel bad? Do you find it makes you feel less worthy and less self-respect? If you do, it is time to realize that giving up can hurt you. It makes one feel awful. It doesn't make you feel better. You will now see that it is more beneficial to persevere through discomfort than to give up. Persisting makes it feel good, and giving in can lead to disappointment.

What about your commitment, drive, and determination? What is keeping you from finding your inner motivation?

Notice the shift in focus away from your goal. How many rewards could you earn if this was your goal? You would feel healthier, slimmer, and more energetic.

Let's redefine this experience. Imagine yourself being able to endure the discomfort, hunger and strain. Imagine completing your plans successfully. Imagine the benefits you could have.

You have all you need in terms of tools, resources, abilities, and knowledge. You should focus on them. If you're committed to your success, it will be obvious how your self-image changes. It feels so empowering. Notice how proud you feel about yourself.

Now, count one through three. One, your work is effortless and easy. You're working as hard or as little as possible. Three, you are seeing the desired results. You are reaching another place, a destination of success. You've achieved your goal.

What does it feel like? Which rewards are you most proud of? Are you more powerful and have better health? Feel the success in you mind and body. Feel the sensation of accomplishment in your mind and body. Imagine being self-disciplined.

Imagine standing firm on solid ground, feeling strong and free. Take a look at the blue sky and you will see the results. Notice how liberated and happy you feel. Notice how success radiates from you.

You might encounter difficulties or disruptions along the way to reaching your goal. You might lose the motivation behind your goal. Then, return to this spot and take a look at the images you see of a new, happy, liberated self.

New opportunities can make you feel excited. Consider them and visualize them as if you were there. Keep your focus on the sense you have of purpose and how it affects how you breathe. Accept the opportunities you have in front of you. Keep this strength with and throughout the day. As you visualize obstacles, boredom, and challenges, imagine yourself walking across them and moving closer to your goal. Grab your hand and touch it. Rewind and look at all the obstacles that have been overcome. How does this make your feel? How proud are you of yourself?

Take a few moments. As you count to three, take this feeling with your. One, you are taking with you the feeling of achievement and success. Look back at the obstacles and realize that you have the strength, capability, and the resources needed to overcome them. Three. You can feel pride and accomplishment, and the awareness about your ability to resist boredom. You feel alert and awake, strong and refreshed. From this point forward, you are confident in your ability keep your eye on the goal. You possess the necessary abilities to accomplish your goal. You are committed in putting your strength, creativity,, and energy into achieving the results you want.

Hypnosis: Enhance Your Self-Image

This hypnosis allows you to release any negative feelings towards yourself. This hypnosis will allow you to get rid of any shame and embarrassment regarding your body or appearance. You will learn to love yourself, be self-respectful, and feel confident.

Take a deep breath and close your eyes. This will help you to shift your beliefs. Be as beautiful in body, mind, & spirit as you can.

Pay attention to what you are doing with your body. Your body holds your beautiful spirit and is infinitely valuable. You should show it the love it deserves. Acceptance and acceptance of your body are key to a higher purpose. Sometimes, it is hard to see your reflection. You'll be amazed at how beautiful and respectable you really are. You will use your mental resources to accomplish this.

Your body acts as your servant. It obeys your orders and acts, tastes, smells, and sees what you ask. It will be easy to fall in love with you. Retire to your chair and close the eyes. You can focus on your heartbeat or the steady rhythm of you breathing. Relax and let your tension go. Allow your body to relax by slowly breathing in and outside. As relaxation sinks deeper, shift your awareness to watch the breathing cycle. Each breath makes you feel more relaxed. You are feeling relaxed and at ease. You are at peace. Follow me to find peaceful relaxation. Feeling good is beneficial for everyone, even if it's difficult. Allow your mind and body to teach you how relax. It is safe to know that you have full control over your life. Imagine yourself crossing an ocean into a world that is safe and peaceful.

Imagine light shining onto you, melting away all tension and warming your soul. It descends onto your head, scanning your brain for negative and painful memories. It replaces them in positive memories and joy. The light fills the body with love and healing energy. It travels to your heart where it dissolves old, painful memories. You are reminded of the endless value in your mind, body, soul. You are in a state of relaxation, letting yourself go, and being able to recover.

The light moves down the body, healing you from pain and suffering. It washes away any painful memories. You can see that your body has become a vessel for the person you always intended to be. It is ready for transformation. Now count down from five minutes to one. Continue relaxing while you count.

At one, you're standing at the end of a bridge which travels into your brain. There you can transform your beliefs to improve self-love/self-respect. You are crossing the bridge. As you move, tension disappears. As you continue to relax, you are eager for a change. At once you are at the entrance of your mind. You can now see the negative emotions, self-loathing and criticism behind you. You have let go. You can see the mirror in front. Look into the mirror. The first impression you get could be painful. It might make you feel less than beautiful or unworthy.

When the mirror is gone, focus on looking inwardly at yourself. You can now see past the mountain of negative emotions. Remember the last moment you saw your authentic self. Create a mirror that shows you the real you. Respect your mirror and show it love. Pay attention to your reflection and you will see the amazing true image of your true selves. You are looking at yourself. Now, look closer and see your true self. See its beauty. You can love yourself just the way that you are. Accepting yourself is part of being you. Respect the real version of yourself.

The true you is a stretch of infinite, which you can see through the mirror. It flows into yourself, exchanging love. You are one and the same as your reflection. Respect and love are what binds you. You're crossing the bridge again to find a source of replenishing and healing water. Drink the fountain to replenish your vessel with love and confidence. Take a look into the water and into your reflection. You can see yourself as you truly are, radiant in health, vitality, love and compassion.

Your true self will be revealed when you take a look at your reflection. You feel self-love, respect, and self-esteem. Now, count to five. At five you will wake yourself up. You will feel deep love and respect towards yourself. You are strong and confident. You can love, respect, and accept your self. Allow the love and acceptance of others, as well as admiration and high esteem, to your body, soul, mind, & body, into your daily life.

Chapter 7: Gastricband Hypnosis –

Weight Loss

It is an understatement when it comes down to weight loss. There is no quick fix or magic bullet. It is a sad fact that almost two thirds (or more) of the world's population are overweight. If there were a simple solution, we would not be where we are today.

Although diet and fitness plans have been heavily promoted, many are seeking out more dramatic solutions to weight issues through gastric bands and stomach sleeve surgeries. The newest player in the weight loss arena is "virtual Gastric Banding" via hypnosis.

Gastric band hypnosis makes the client hypnotize and suggests that they have been through a lapbanding operation. This is meant to assist them with portion control in an observant environment.

Some hypnotherapists charge over $1,000 for weekend-group sessions. But, although virtual gastrointestinal methods are becoming more popular, experts say that hypnosis in weight loss is not new.

What's it all about? So, what's the deal? Are you satisfied? Is it successful? How can you navigate a market that is relatively unregulated without losing your interest in hypnotherapy?

What is Hypnosis exactly?

This is the process of deep relaxation. These methods are not unique; many cultures have used them for thousands upon thousands ofyears.

This therapy has become increasingly popular for treating anxiety, panic disorder, depression and sleep issues.

This treatment is also known by the name hypnotherapy.

There are no other expectations that can be placed on the individual, despite what trashy TV shows might tell you. The individual is fully in control. Hypnosis does not force anyone to do something they don't want to. It's voluntary. It's voluntary society.

Hypnosis really works to lose weight?

Mailin Colman, president Australian Hypnotherapists Association - AHA says that hypnosis can be a great option for anyone looking to lose weight. However the virtual lap banding option may not work for everyone.

The virtual lap band (Virtual Lap Bands) has been around for years. While they can work well for some people, weight loss can be hard because everyone's motivations and causes of eating and overeating can be very diverse. You can have a good hypnotherapist work with you to identify the root causes of your problems. "There are many strategies that work for different clients," she states. Clare Collins is spokesperson for Dietitian Association of Australia (DAA). She says that there are not many studies on hypnosis. This she believes shows a "disconnection between theory, practice and theory." She claimed that experiments have had mixed success in the past, and they are difficult to perform because blind subjects are not able to do them.

She stated that an extensive analysis of the previous work and findings presented by Liverpool John Moores University in 2014. was performed to analyze it. Overall, the study revealed that some people can benefit from weight-loss hypnosis when it's used in conjunction with conventional weight-control methods and is regularly implemented (not just one-off). The study did show that hypnosis didn't work for all people. Hypnosis only worked well in those who were open-minded and hypnotic.

Multi-pronged strategy is the best

Collins says that hypnosis will help those who react well. It can deal with negative self communications and self-sabotage.

Collins insists that hypnosis alone is not enough. Collins states that "hypnosis alone is not sufficient. There are cognitive behavioral therapies, which may be more effective for people than hypnosis. But it is important to understand healthy eating and exercise habits.

He explained that many people are tempted to just go for the quickest fix, rather than undergoing a comprehensive nutritional assessment.

"Weightloss is so difficult that it's impossible to lose weight, so you have to approach it with different points of views in order achieve your goals. Exercise and diet are important, but it's also important to take into consideration psychological factors. She says that it is equally important for people to understand the reasons behind being overweight.

Collins explained that it is possible to have therapy with a counselor, who can combine techniques like relaxation. "Even though patients may want lap band surgery, there are often waiting lists. In these cases, I suggest that patients try other options to help them succeed while they wait.

It is important to recognize that there is no regulation in this industry. Anyone can start a shop claiming to be a hypnotherapist.

Here are some professional suggestions:

* Make sure the hypnotherapist joins an association. Australian Society and Australian Hypnotherapy Association, which are the two largest, require members to receive supervision, regular training, minimal training requirements and professional experience.

* Accreditation is often granted by organizations based on research and expertise. ASCH professionals can work as dentists, doctors, psychologists, or chiropractors. The AHA monitors participants at different levels. This includes teachers, practitioners, and clinicians. Clinical members spend at least 500 hours with clients.

* You should ensure that your first-aid nurses have a credential.

* Many private training schools with accreditation from the government for hypnotherapists. There are many websites that provide information.

* Make sure you find a hypnotherapist that has additional skills. Many have worked as advisers or studied to become hypnotherapists. Some psychologists have hypnotherapy as a part of their practice.

Register online. ASCH and AHA list hypnotherapists. There you can verify the individual qualifications. Ask your therapist any questions regarding their training and past experience.

* Many medical plans offer discounts to therapists who practice hypnotherapy. Be sure to verify before you book.

* Contact the hypnotherapist by phone or in person before scheduling a paid consultation appointment. This allows you test your credentials as well as to feel the therapist, if you're a good listener.

* Prices are important. Although there is no official schedule for practitioners' fees, the range between $100 and $250

per hour is a reasonable estimate. Colman stated that she believes anything higher than $250 is unacceptable and should be flagged by potential customers.

* How many sessions do your sessions consist of? This could be similar to asking the length of a string. It depends on what you're being treated for. Our experts advise that you check with another person if you don't feel comfortable being treated by your therapist in the first session. Colman suggests that the consumer will see improvement after three sessions.

Sally of Queensland: Case Study

Sally states that she was attracted to virtual gastric blnging because it seemed to be a less "drastic" solution than real gastric blnging.

She states that her weight gain was a problem for quite some time. She suggested the possibility of a gastric lap band procedure. She claims that she was looking for the hypnosis version and came across them during her studies.

Sally stated that she approached a hypnotherapist within her city. He said that he had done virtual gastric bandsage and arranged to meet with her. However, she says that she didn't test for any therapists before choosing one.

She said that she paid $200 extra to have the hypnotherapist sit on a cushioned chair with a blanket. They then started talking about a soundtrack which featured the sounds of an operating-room.

Sally was a nurse and almost couldn't settle down because the music in her hospital wasn't perfect. She also claimed that the nurse was reading from a familiar script. She also claimed that the sound was not the right one, but that it was the correct computer. She was also shocked to learn that he had not spoken to her about her personal circumstances before the hypnosis. "He never asked me any questions about me, about how I lost weight, or about what my mission was." He didn't even say anything. Sally received a new soundtrack CD to listen to at home after her sessions, and was instructed to return for further sessions. She states that she didn't prefer it as she "essentially didn't feel anything else" and didn't realize how it helped.

She told me she was disappointed that she paid $200 to have her approach tailored to her particular needs. "It could have tried something else if gastric banding did not work. It felt very one-size fits most.

Are Weight Loss Hypnosis and Hypnosis Really Effective?

If you are part of a diet, exercise, therapy weight-loss program, weight losshypnosis can help motivate you to shed another pound. Because there are not enough reliable scientific data for hypnosis, it can be difficult to determine if this is a positive weight loss.

Hypnosis, a state that allows you to relax and concentrate mentally, is similar to being in a trance. Hypnosis involves the use of visual imagery and verbal repetition with a trained hypnotherapist.

Under hypnosis, you have a strong focus and respond well to suggestions.

Some studies looked into the possibility of weight loss using hypnosis. Research showed that weight loss was minimal. In fact, the average weight loss in 18-months was only 6 pounds (2,7kg). However, these researches are not necessarily valid and it is difficult to say if weight reduction hypnosis has validity.

However, a recent study which only showed marginal results in weight reduction found that patients receiving hypnosis had lower inflammation, greater happiness, and a better quality of life. There could be other factors that influence weight with hypnosis. Further research is needed to fully understand the possible weight loss effects of hypnosis.

A combination of diet and exercise is the best way to lose weight. If you have tried exercise and diet but are still not achieving your weight loss goals, you should talk to your physician about what other lifestyle options you may be able to make.

The weight loss hypnosis does not guarantee dramatic weight loss. But, for certain people it might be worth trying along with a lifestyle change.

What Gastric Band Surgery can you do to lose weight?

There are many options available if your doctor has agreed that the weight-loss procedure is appropriate for your needs. A surgeon uses several techniques to reduce your stomach size in a restrictive procedure. Restrictive treatment allows you to move better and eat less.

The full names for these three styles of weight loss restrictive operations are:

* Flexible gastric bands for laparoscopy

* Vertical gastroplasty bandsage

* Sleeve-gastrectomy

What Does Gastric Banding Surgery Actually Mean?

The surgeon uses laparoscopy, which involves making small cuts in one's stomach. The silicone band squeezes out the stomach, transforming it into a pouch that measures approximately one inch. After banding the stomach, it can hold just one ounce.

A plastic tube runs from the silicone belt to the underlying unit. The silicone band can be opened and closed with saline. Injecting saline will fill and tighten the unit. This helps to tighten or loosen the band, which can help to reduce side effects.

What are the Gastric Banding Recommendations?

Due to its high success rate, gastric bands are no longer common. This treatment can result in weight loss of approximately 35% to 45%. One example is someone who is more than 100 lbs might lose 35 to 45lbs after gastric bandsing. However, these results are not always consistent. The stomach can usually return to normal size if it is necessary.

What are the consequences for gastric banding

Gastric Banding is very easy for most people. Gastric banding does not pose any risk of death. These are the main problems with gastric surgery.

* Nausea, vomiting and constipation are two of the most common side effects after gastric bandsing. This can sometimes be reduced by loosening the band.

* Mild complications during surgery. These include minor bleeding, adjustment problems and injury infections.

Gastric banding doesn't interfere with food absorption, as opposed to gastric bypass. It is rare to develop vitamin deficiencies after gastric surgery. However, approximately half of your stomach will be removed during a Sleeve Gastrectomy. You'll still have a thin, vertical sleeve the size of a banana. The surgery isn't reversible as part of your stomach will be removed.

What Does Sleeve Gastrectomy Actually Mean?

Due to its success rate as well as the low number of complications, gastric surgery has become one of the most preferred restrictive operations. People who had this operation reported losing 40- 50% of their body weight.

The operation can either be performed through a large incision made in the abdomen (open procedure) or via laparoscopically with several small incisions that use small instruments and a guide camera. Physical recovery takes approximately 4 to 6 week.

What is Gastroplasty Vertical Banded?

The VBG also has a plastic band placed around the stomach. Also, the surgeon placed the stomach in a tight pocket and covered it with the band.

Vertical banding gastroplasty produces a higher weight loss than any other operation. There is also a higher chance of confusion. Vertical gastroplasty today is less common. This procedure is performed by only 5 percent of bariatric surgery surgeons.

What is Mixed Surgery and How Does It Work?

Malabsorptive and restrictive surgery are important parts of every weight loss procedure. A typical weight-loss procedure includes restrictive surgery. The "stomach button" is used to create a tiny stomach pocket. The new stomach bag is then attached to a section of the smallintestine. This causes lower food consumption and food absorption (malabsorptive).

Chapter 8: Virtual Gastric Box

Hyponosis

A virtual stomach band is a method that qualified hypnotists use to indicate that you are wearing a gastric tube around your abdomen. Gastric hypnotherapy will guide you through virtual surgery planning, virtual procedure, as well as a safe and comfortable postoperative lifestyle.

The treatment does not involve any procedures or medicines and it is completely non-invasive. Many people who have had the simulated operation felt more full after eating than they did during a real procedure.

Actual gastric band surgery

This surgery is recommended for obese patients who weigh more than 45kg and have not been able to lose weight.

The gastric bypass procedure involves the placement of a band on the stomach. It will reduce the amount of food a person is allowed to eat. You will eat less and run faster, which helps you lose fat.

This is an operation which can involve risks and complications.

* Post-operative infections

* Lung or deadly injured leg or lung blood Clots

* Internal bleeding

* Troubles with diarrhoea or reflux

How does it work?

Surgery can be a significant decision for anyone. This is especially true if you are overweight. The benefits of hypnosis to the gastric system are innumerable. The objective is to accept that your stomach has decreased in size and that you were able to have the operation done clinically at an unconscious level.

The hypnotherapist uses proven methods to help you enter hypnosis. However, you will always be in control of the events around you. You will not be awake or asleep, so you cannot do something you don't want to.

The sub-conscious mind at this comfortable point is open to suggestions from the therapist concerning your weight loss goals.

The most important aspect of treatment for the virtual gastric bypass would then be performed by the hypnotherapist. It will be possible to receive powerful reminders that you can mount a virtual gastric band.

Virtual Gastric Band for me?

The mind is very powerful. While you might not realize it, at a conscious level, you will see that there is no specific procedure. However, if you subconsciously accept that your physical gastric bands was activated and support the recommendations regarding planning before and after surgery, then it is probable that it will work.

Gastric bandhypnosis requires a lot of commitment. The more you treat it like a gastric bypass procedure, the better it will be. You will always have the ability to make mistakes, and you can exercise your free will.

Healthy living is the result everyday decisions, healthy eating habits, changes in lifestyle.

Maximize the Process

The results of hypnotherapy virtual gaztric band depend on how strongly you believe in the process as well as the abilities of your therapist.

A key component of any hypnosis therapy is the confidence that the hypnotherapist works well for you.

If you want to lose weight, the virtual gastric bypass offers real hope. To be able to succeed and take the next step, it is necessary to make lifestyle changes that will allow you to live a full life.

GASTRICBAND HYPNOSIS TO FOOD ADDICTION

Is there any hypnosis that can be used to stop binging? It works only for eating disorders such as overeating or unhealthy eating.

Do you ever feel your life is all about food and drink?

Food is an integral part in our daily lives.

But, food is something we've been taught to dislike. We've been taught to eat food. And many of us hunt for sugar. They eat food when they feel stressed. Others seek unrestricted indulgence. Others turn to food when bored.

The explanation is straightforward: Our subconscious prepares food to be used as a security cupboard.

That's right. That's why we want to feel secure in the subconscious. This vast knowledge store governs 85-95% all of our thoughts. The fight-or–flight response is an unconscious natural defense mechanism. It protects us when we are in danger.

When we succumb the sugar temptations, our subconscious is in a defensive mode. It is because of this that we feel compelled to snack or eat more immediately. Our subconscious knows succulent snacks or feeling overwhelmed mean 'health.' In other words: Overcoming food addiction requires more than willpower. You heard it right. There is no need to become addicted to food. The trick is to teach your subconscious mind how to accept these subconscious-cravings, and then let them go.

That's why food addiction hypnosis can prove so effective.

Hypnosis provides access to the subconscious. Communicating with the subconscious clearly will help us to get rid of our bad habits and train it as a supporter. It's actually simpler than it appears.

Perhaps you are wondering how hypnosis works for food addiction. You may think something like this about it: Hypnosis opens the door to a direct line of communication with your subconscious. We can have constructive statements, new knowledge and direct communication with the subconscious. Hypnosis could reprogram your consciousness.

What is Food Addiction (FA)?

Food addiction is a medical term that can lead to a wide range of unhealthy food relationships.

Binge eating disorder, for example, is when people eat large quantities of food. Binge eating occurs when someone eats in short periods of time, sometimes slowly and can consume thousands of calories. These binges can have serious health effects. Binge eating can be overwhelming. Hypnosis is a method that allows you to control and regulate your binging impulses.

Compulsive Overeating is another example. Compulsive food overeating causes a lot of cravings. They are most often compelled to eat sugars, milk and carbs. According to National Center for Eating Disorders, they are unable to control their cravings. Hypnosis helps to understand fears and reprogram unconscious thoughts to overcome impulses.

Others are known to be sugar addicts and carb addicts. Their cravings for particular foods do not seem to stop them from eating more of these unhealthy meals. Sugar addiction therapy, for example, can help to change the way our subconscious perceives sugar and help us feel satisfied.

No matter the type of dependence, many addicts experience similar symptoms.

* Eating quickly

* You should eat even when you are full

* Eating discreetly, even when you're not hungry

* Secret eating

* Feeling shame and guilt for overeating

* Feeling compelled, "oriented" to eat.

Subconsciousness is where the roots of food addiction lie. Our subconscious minds have been trained to associate good with certain food types, like overeating and binging.

How our Thoughts Can Help Food Addictions

It is not the overcrowding of binging and extreme cravings that are the problem. Instead, it is our negative thinking patterns which lead us to make unhealthy food decisions.

Such connections are deeply rooted. We've spent our entire lives trying to make ourselves safe to eat.

Parties, parties and grandma baking cookies - we've found that our mates are fond of delicious foods as well as unhealthy food. Many of us use it as a way to relax, relieve boredom, or anxiety, and others for food.

It is very common for our cravings to be accidentally activated. BAM! We feel pain! We just go to work and eat, without ever really thinking about why.

Sometimes our subconscious minds aren't even known. Evidence indicates that 85-95% if brain activity takes place there. This is the brain region that causes food dependence.

The subconscious impulses that drive us are innate and have been reinforced by our lifetime of experience. One example is that after a traumatic childhood, we might have found comfort and relief in food. This may help us replace feelings of shame or hurt. As you can clearly see, we can transform to ease our pain.

You may also have good moments that are related to your hunger. Imagine: Sweets are synonymous with grandma baking. Sweets are in fact connected to love or comfort in their subconsciousness. This is the reason why so many people turn towards emotional food or stress - they want to be comforted.

The good news about the subconscious is that it can be retrained. Hypnosis is a way to naturally and efficiently rely on our subconscious. These symptoms, including anxiety and stress, can also be caused by dysfunctional thinking habits.

Hypnosis is a way to become hyper-conscious of your hunger. We learn to accept them. These happen all the time, often instinctively, and sometimes without thought. But once we recognize them, our hunger can be overcome.

Hypnosis is also a way to reach the subconscious and transmit new, more valuable knowledge to this immense repository of knowledge. It is like removing weeds to plant new seeds. We must change how we view fast food.

GASTRICBAND HYPONOSIS FOOD ADDICTION: HOW ITS WORKS

I think you have an idea about why hypnosis works. Hypnosis makes us aware of our needs, and teaches us how we should approach food. How does it all work?

Here are some examples of fine hypnosis for food dependency, and the many ways it can help us lead healthier lives.

* Mindful Eating. Almost all food habits share a similar symptom. It has become a habit so that we don't think about the consequences. By hypnosis, mindful eating will teach the mind how to recognize our hunger and what it means for us. Hypnosis with careful food allows one to identify cravings, physical symptoms of hunger, and become more aware about what you eat. We take control of our food intake and thirst.

* Breaking out of the Normal: All too often our normal thinking is negative and pessimistic. These thoughts can cause us to crave food or overeat. In stressful situations at work, you may find yourself worrying about your ability to breathe and say everything is fine. Without increasing spiraling thoughts, we cannot get rid of our food addictions. Hypnosis aids us in regaining control of our thoughts.

* Resolving the Reasons behind it: An addiction to food can be caused many ways: stress, anxiety and lack of self love. Hypnosis allows us to manage these conditions and move past them.

* Restoring Trust. A lack of trust or affection won't allow us to act. If we lack trust in ourselves and respect ourselves, our bad behaviors will not change. Hypnotherapy offers a strong way to build trust in yourself and to develop compassion. This is important for people who have food addictions. If

we love ourselves and believe that we are worthy, we can confront hunger and choose to live a healthy life.

Self-Hypnosis for Overcoming Bad or Unhealthy Eating Habits

There are several options available for individuals in hypnotherapy. These include one-on-1 consultations with a trained hypnotherapist and videos of self-hypnosis. Self-hypnosis offers convenience as it can be done from home or at work.

It is strongly advised for people suffering from food addictions. Grace's selfhypnosis tutorial will help you. It is easy as pie. Here are some things you might want:

* Be mindful of your well being: How do you feel about yourself? It is important to assess how you feel at the end of each session.

* Guided meditation/visualization: Deep breaths indicate to the body and mind that relaxation is possible. Another way to calm is visualization.

* A Guided Counterdown: You may choose to count down 10 or more. It allows you to hypnose your mind.

* Positive affirmations - You will communicate your thoughts to the subconscious even if you are not at home. For a mind-remodeling effect, provide facts and positive ideas. Perhaps you say, "I'm free of overeating and food addiction." I hear my body asking me what to eat. Balanced foods are best for me. I stop sweetening food. Each day, I feel better...

* Visualization for Change: Visualize your safer path after making your unconscious constructive suggestions. A balanced food partnership is possible. It helps the concept to grow and supports itself.

Hypnotherapy or Aversion Therapy: Reframing You Mind

Side effects from salty, fatty or sweet foods include many. Overindulgence is linked to obesity and diabetes, energy scarcity, depression, and other health problems. It causes lower productivity, anxiety, and increased sexy desire. These foods are necessary to survive.

How could we make it so that the mind doesn't crave unhealthy food? Even if I didn't see a brownie, or chocolate cake, my mind wouldn't believe that I should.

Hypnosis for avoidance, which is a technique that hypnotherapists are trained in, can be very beneficial to us. It's not always essential, but it is one of most successful ways to treat food addiction.

We aren't huge fans of aversion treatment for most subjects. However when it is about food and sugar, aversion Therapy can be so successful for tipping consumer scales that they have to include it in this post. (What we want to see is a lean healthy body rather that a negative copy of what they don't, like a cake with ants).

Aversion therapy helps you to identify with the bad while also helping you make constructive connections for the best decision. A hypnotherapist could start by saying food is life. Food is natural and comes directly from nature. Agriculture.

They could then build a misleading junkfood association, meaning that the food is potentially harmful or even deadly to our bodies.

You should remember that our subconscious must make it feel liberated. Because of this, when we eat juice boxes and other fatty snacks, it assumes that we have been given a favor. But it didn't. But it didn't.

Why not for the subconscious? Don't view junk food in a way that rewards you or gives you safety, but as a dangerous choice.

Gastric Band Hypnosis for Food Addiction - Does it work?

What the research says

The majority of research has been conducted in the area of hypnosis for food cravings or sugar loss. The process is straightforward. It has been proven that Hypnosis is a powerful tool for helping people lose their weight.

In fact, a study found that people who had hypnosis reported suffering 20 percent more than those with no hypnosis. Many studies have also shown that hypnosis to promote healthy eating leads to more lasting results.

- Weight Loss: In 1986 researchers studied how hypnosis might help 60 people lose their weight. Participants used hypnosis for self-improvement, decision making and inspiration. In hypnosis groups, participants lost on average 30 times as much, or 17 to 0.25 pounds.

- Participants in Hypnosis Last over 90% of Others: This meta-analysis was performed relative to cognitive behavior therapy. It included 18 studies that examined hypnosis and weight loss. Relaxation training, directed visualization and other similar treatments were compared to those that were enhanced by hypnosis. The results: hypnosis resulted is weight loss and weight decrease. The hypnosis-users lost over 90% of non-hypnosis people and kept it off until two years later.

- Long-term weight loss: One study examined the effects of hypnosis on the therapeutic weight management system. The study included 109 participants. All the participants lost significant weight within nine weeks. However, both the eight-month-old and the two-year-old following the incident, the hypnosis communities continued to lose weight and reached their weight goals.

GASTRIC-BAND HYPONOSIS OVERVIEW

A gastricband is a flexible silicone silicone device that aids in weight loss. The strip is placed on the upper stomach area to form a small pouch. This reduces the amount food that can be processed and makes it less difficult to eat large quantities.

A gastric Band is used to reduce food intake to induce weight loss. The procedure is only for people who have tried other methods to lose weight. Like all surgeries, there are risks.

Gastric band-hypnosis can help people lose weight naturally without any complications. Many hypnotherapists will use gastric bandhypnosis. This is a two-way process. First, determine what is causing your emotional eating.

The therapist will assist you in recollecting long forgotten memories regarding food. Before you can perform hypnotherapy to the stomach band, it is helpful to address and recognize unhealthy food thought patterns.

The hypnotherapist then should take charge of the virtual unit. This technique is meant to signal that you had an operation in which a gastric tube was placed at an unconscious stage. The idea is that your body will feel better and it will act as if you were actually doing something.

These systems can be followed for a short time, but may not be as effective over the long term. Many diets require us to count calories, or have portions measured or exclude certain types of foods. This can lead to increased food and health concerns.

How Gastric Band Hypnosis Functions

Hypnotists place you in a state known as hypnosis by using relaxation techniques. Your subconscious will be more open to suggestion when you are relaxed. This is when hypnotherapists are able to make suggestions to you subconscious. This is what gastric band therapy does.

The mind is powerful. Your actions will change if you follow these suggestions subconsciously. Most often, the virtual gastric units are accompanied with ideas about trust, and actions that can help you make lifestyle changes.

Many therapists will also help you to learn self-hypnosis techniques in order to build on the research that was done during the session. It is also recommended to educate yourself about diet, exercise, and other topics that can help promote health and wellbeing.

The Processes

You will meet the hypnotherapist for the first time in a consultation. In this session, you will learn more about what hypnotherapy has to offer. This is a time to discuss past attempts at weight loss, dietary habits, health issues, and general food preferences. This knowledge helps the psychiatrist to understand what works, and whether or not other types of therapy are possible.

The method is intended to make gastric surgery look like it really did. Many hypnotherapists will add the sounds, smells and sights of operating rooms to make the experience more authentic. Your therapist should begin by getting you to a deeply relaxed state. It is sometimes called hypnosis. You will be aware and in control of all that is happening.

The therapist will talk to patients during surgery when they are in this state. I will take you through the steps, from the anesthesia to the first incision, to the band and how to heal the wound. It should be easy to relax and feel at ease in the operating room.

You can make additional interventions to boost self-confidence as part of the process, as mentioned above. After you are done, your hypnotherapist might teach you some self-hypnosis techniques to help you track where you are at all times.

Some hypnotherapists might recommend that your return to follow-up appointments be held to assess the progress of the virtual band, and to make any necessary adjustments. This is done when people are also fitted in the physical band. For some, hypnotherapy sessions might be beneficial as part long-term weight management programs. This is a great way for the hypnotherapist, to work with your to address your self-esteem and underlying diet issues.

Include gastric band therapy in your diet and exercise plans. It is common to lose weight by changing your habits in both your body as well as your mind.

How/What do I Feel After I Do?

Gastric band therapy is designed to promote healthy eating habits. If your subconscious perceives you have gastric bands attached, your stomach might feel smaller. This sends your brain messages telling you that you are full after eating fewer calories.

It can be difficult to identify when you're full for those who eat too much. Sometimes we eat for comfort or our pleasure and don't recognize if we're actually hungry. To be able to better understand hunger and fullness, you will need to adopt healthier eating habits.

Contrary gastric band surgeries, virtual gastric bands do not have any side effects. Some people may experience nausea, vomiting or acid reflux after true surgery. Such symptoms are rare because gastric bandhypnosis can't be performed.

The treatment process will be fun and relaxing. Most people feel hypnotized.

Is This Going To Work for Me?

Many people who have tried hypnotherapy for the first time ask this question: "Does it work?" Unfortunately, it is not as simple as a yes or no. Most of it is yours. Hypnotherapy has many benefits, but it's especially effective in changing behavior. This is why many people find success in changing their eating habits and losing weight. This weight loss program requires dedication and commitment, just as any other.

Gastric band Hypnotherapy is more successful if you are able to trust your therapist as well as the method. It is essential to feel comfortable and confident with your hypnotherapist. It is important to take the time and research hypnotherapists within your field. Learn about their methods and skills. Before the procedure, you can ensure that they are comfortable with you.

If you are looking to make a change in your life and can trust your hypnotherapist for guidance, gastric band therapy may be right for you.

Gastric Band Hypnosis - What you do not know